AF883570

CHALLENGING ATTACHMENT THEORY

Drawing on decades of cross-cultural research, Heidi Keller reveals how attachment theory is rooted in WEIRD societies representing less than 10% of humanity, despite claims to universality. Through rigorous analysis, she systematically deconstructs core assumptions, demonstrating how a culturally specific model has been inappropriately universalized and exposing fundamental scientific flaws.

Keller presents compelling ethnographic evidence from diverse cultural communities, revealing multiple valid pathways to forming secure relationships that attachment theory fails to recognize. She shows how feeding practices, cultural learning, and community-based caregiving create strong bonds that don't fit the Western dyadic mother–child model. Beyond theoretical critique, she examines the real-world consequences of attachment theory's dominance in parenting interventions across the Global South, family court custody decisions, and early childhood education programs, demonstrating how these applications, presented as evidence-based, often pathologize non-WEIRD parenting practices and impose inappropriate standards on diverse families.

This groundbreaking work calls for nothing less than the decolonization of developmental science, advocating for culturally conscious research that respects local knowledge, embraces methodological diversity, and abandons the search for universal developmental pathways. Keller provides concrete steps toward achieving truly inclusive and ethical research practices that honor the full spectrum of human development. Essential reading for researchers, practitioners, and policymakers in child development, education, social work, and international development – a transformative analysis that will fundamentally reshape your understanding of child development and culture.

Heidi Keller is Professor Emeritus of Psychology and former Head of Department, Culture and Development, Faculty of Human Sciences, Osnabrueck University, Germany. Among many international awards, in 2019 she was the recipient of the SRCD Award for Distinguished Contributions to Understanding International, Cultural and Contextual Diversity in Child Development.

'This book is a *tour de force*, wherein Keller shares her conceptual brilliance and knowledge in informative and entertaining ways. It is an essential aid in increasing inclusivity and decreasing colonial practices in how we interact with children and families. Amid constructive criticism of current theory and practice in developmental psychology (rightly characterized as WEIRD, pertaining to mostly Western middle-income contexts), Keller brings illuminating descriptions of children developing within a wide variety of ecocultural contexts around the world. I can easily conceive of this book as becoming integral in the education of university students, of Ethics Review Boards, and of practitioners, from pediatricians to teachers, from those providing parenting advice to those providing early interventions. This book is an exemplary presentation of the need for and benefits of viewing childhood within ecocultural context.'

Prof. Dr. Kim A. Bard, ***Professor of Comparative Developmental Psychology, Affiliate Scientist, University of Michigan-Dearborn, USA***

'This is a book that begins with life and compels theory to respond. Emerging from a trajectory that moves from kitchens to communities, from observation to uneasy understanding, it unsettles the long-standing assumption that culture is a variable to be added to psychological models. Here, culture appears as the very ground of perception, the condition through which development becomes intelligible.

What gives this work its force is its engagement with diverse childhoods across contexts and its methodological honesty. The recognition that not knowing language, misreading practices, and depending on others are not limitations to be overcome, but conditions that reshape what it means to know. In this sense, the book offers a rare account of how psychological knowledge is actually made through relationships, mistakes, and sustained encounters with difference.

Its return to attachment theory is particularly significant. Rather than accepting or dismissing it, the author approaches it as an ethical problem, one that must be confronted in light of the many childhoods that lie outside its assumptions. This is not critique for its own sake, but an insistence that widely accepted frameworks be made answerable to the worlds they claim to describe.

Situated within ongoing efforts to decolonize psychology, this book does something more demanding: it does not simply call for change, but demonstrates how such change emerges from a lifetime of engagement with people, practices, and places that resist easy translation. It will be of interest not only to developmental psychologists but also to anyone concerned with how knowledge travels, transforms, and sometimes fails.'

Prof. Dr. Nandita Chaudhary, ***Professor in the Department of Cultural Psychology, Federal University of Bahia, Salvador da Bahia***

CHALLENGING ATTACHMENT THEORY

Ethnocentrism, Science, and Child Development

Heidi Keller

Routledge
Taylor & Francis Group
LONDON AND NEW YORK

Designed cover image: Other, Heidi Keller

First published 2027
by Routledge
4 Park Square, Milton Park, Abingdon, Oxon OX14 4RN

and by Routledge
605 Third Avenue, New York, NY 10158

Routledge is an imprint of the Taylor & Francis Group, an informa business

British Library Cataloguing-in-Publication Data
A catalogue record for this book is available from the British Library

ISBN: 9781041138990 (hbk)
ISBN: 9781041138983 (pbk)
ISBN: 9781003672050 (ebk)

DOI: 10.4324/9781003672050

Typeset in Sabon
by codeMantra

CONTENTS

A PERSONAL PREFACE

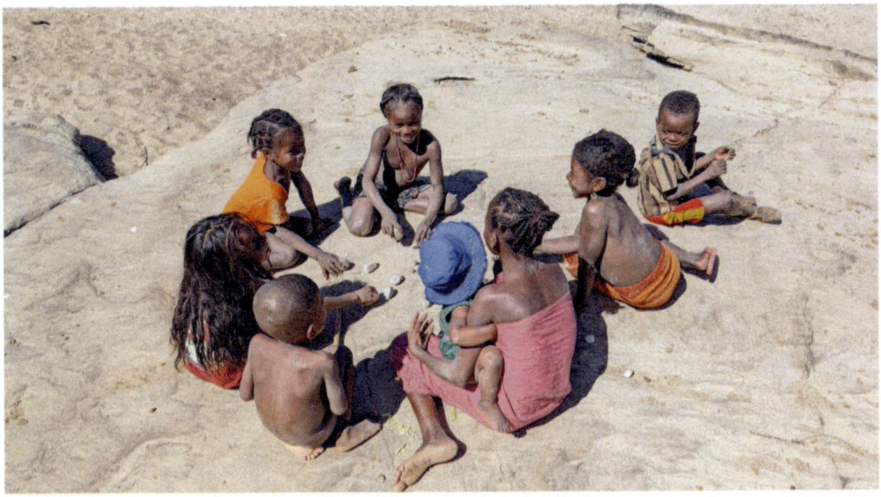

FIGURE 1 Children in Menamaty, southern Madagascar. Copyright Gabriel Scheidecker

The development of research interests is part of individual biographies. Biographies are diverse, as are research interests, which is vividly documented in Frank Kessel's *Pillars of Developmental Psychology* (2025). Frank Kessel has invited 40 present developmental psychologists to write essays about how they became who they are. These essays are exemplary in demonstrating diversity, not only in interests and career pathways but also in writing styles and emphases. My personal scientific story took many random turns. It all started with my interest in other cultures. From childhood on, I was fascinated by other countries, the diversity of food, and landscapes. My first book consequently became a cookbook. Together with my friend from Barbados, Miranda Greaves, I wrote a cookbook about Caribbean Kitchen, which first appeared in 1988. We did not want to disseminate just recipes, but also the stories about the food and the dishes. My interest in these dimensions of culture never vanished but became part of a general curiosity about the diversity of life and culture as the pervasive environment of human development. I understood that culture is not located in museums and theaters as an interesting addition to life, a dimension or a variable, as it is still conceived in many parts of psychology until today, but the foundation of existence and the glasses through which we look into the world.

The content of my scientific interests was for a long time children's development in different cultures. I wanted to understand how children grow up in diverse environments and what the similarities and differences are. With a minor in ethology, I was trained in observational methods. Observing babies in villages in the Northwest of Cameroon or Indian Gujarat told me very fast that children's development across cultures cannot be understood in terms of one model with more or less, earlier or later. Children develop differently in different environments, nevertheless addressing similar developmental tasks. One of the major communalities of children's development is the centrality of social relationships. I was fascinated by the different care arrangements, different social environments, and also the different physical set-ups in which children can be found and social life is situated. My curiosity about why different communities raised children the way they did prevented me from taking my own template as the standard. However, observations were not enough; I wanted to know why babies were cared for the way they were. Not knowing the local languages and the local communication rules was a big challenge and the best training in recognizing pitfalls and bias in cross-cultural methodology. Starting from scratch and not using existing instruments like scales or questionnaires necessitates listening to people's voices. Not understanding the local language means first establishing a collaboration network as an utmost necessity. This means developing mutually trusting relationships, based on knowledge and respect for local customs, communication rules, and modes of conduct. Lots of opportunities to make mistakes ...

All these experiences brought me back to attachment theory, with which I had a long history of avoidance. I encountered attachment theory at its beginnings in Germany through Klaus and Karin Großmann. The group of scholars interested in infants and infancy in Germany at that time, the 1970s, was more than manageable. Babies were considered not to be scientific subject, and observation methodology was a career killer. Thus, joining the Grossmann group (Klaus Großmann was already an established professor) and becoming an attachment researcher would have been the best option for an early-career scholar. However, I had reservations against attachment theory from the beginning. I thought the Strange Situation Procedure was unethical, putting small children into despair, as I could observe in labs in the United States. I saw the incongruities and fuzziness of the theory and the closeness of the attachment circle, not considering any of the criticisms that were there right from the beginning. After having seen the different realities of many babies in the Global South, I decided that avoidance is not a scientific attitude and that helping to put attachment theory in its place is an ethical necessity.

Once alerted, more and more issues came up that led to deep unease about just continuing on a sidetrack in a parallel scientific world. I was happy enough to meet colleagues from all over the world who shared the same urge to work for a change, to work for the decolonization of psychological theories and methods. I want to particularly thank Kim Bard, Nandita Chaudhary, and Gabriel Scheidecker, with whom I have collaborated closely over the last few years in different projects. Without them, this book could never have been written.

Heidi Keller
Deuselbach, April 2026.

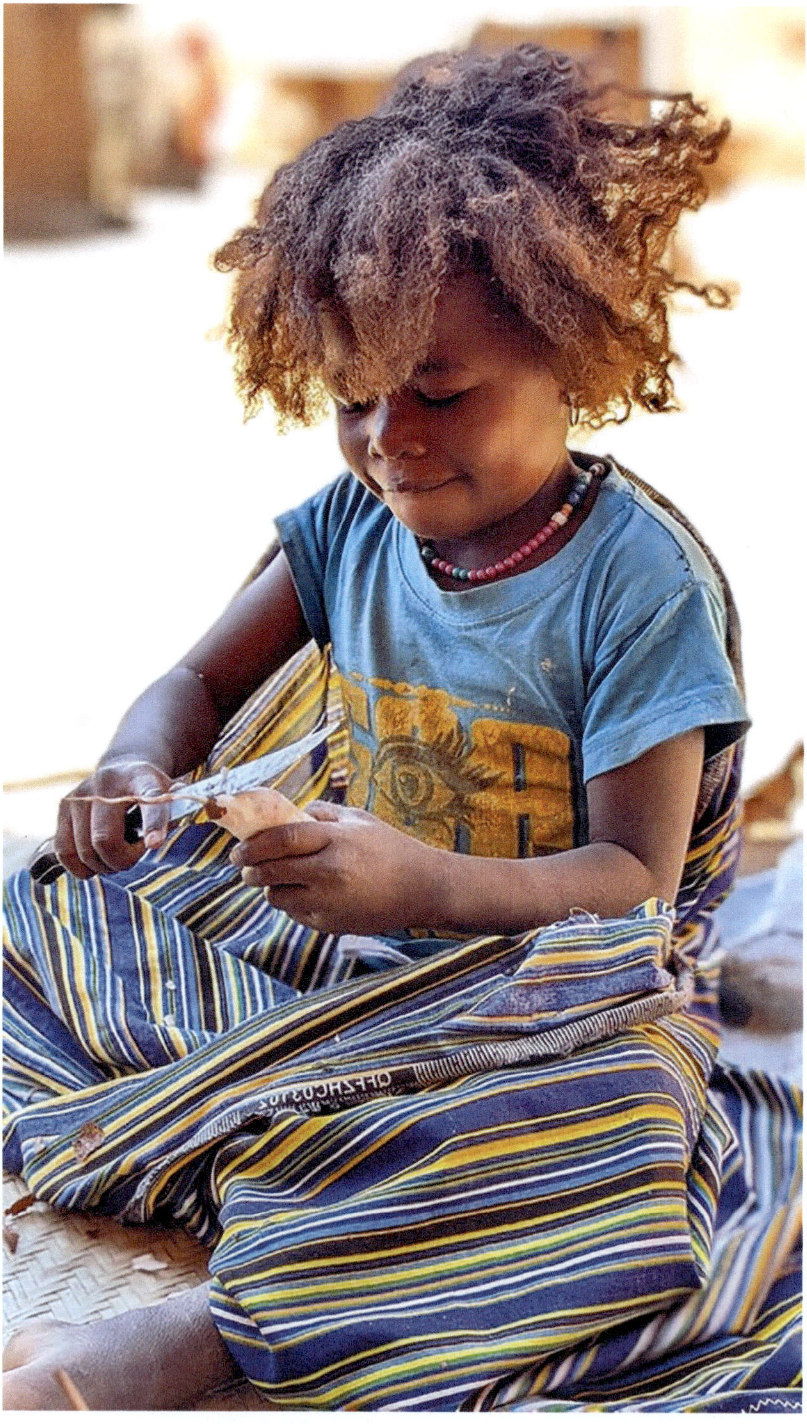

FIGURE 2 Child in Menamaty, southern Madagascar. Copyright Gabriel Scheidecker

PART 1

Setting the stage

1

WHO IS PSYCHOLOGY ABOUT?

Abstract

This chapter deals with the providers of knowledge in psychology and the social sciences in general: the person, the participant in research studies. It is argued that a universal participant is proclaimed in mainstream psychology, which necessarily marginalizes the individual and the context. The universal participant belongs to the Western middle class because of the predominance of Western middle-class researchers, mainly capitalizing on convenience samples, i.e., Western middle-class participants. Nevertheless, there is also variation among Western middle-class samples that is equally ignored. This procedure results in interpreting research results in generic terms, assuming universal validity. It is argued that contextualizing participants is necessary to understand who provides research evidence and to whom it possibly applies.

Psychology aims to understand and explain how individuals think, feel, and act. As an empirical science, its knowledge base is created with and from people, the participants in research studies. Yet there is generally not much attention devoted to who these people are. Samples are mainly characterized by the number of participants, their age, and eventually also the gender distribution.

Results are presented in generic terms, implying that they are valid across people and contexts so that the composition of samples is negligible. In other words, persons seem to be interchangeable because a single human prototype is assumed. The consequence is convenience samples, with mainly university students as the most accessible group being overrepresented. Besides the fact

DOI: 10.4324/9781003672050-2

that university students are one small part of societies and cultures that have more similarities across countries and cultures than other pockets of society (e.g., higher formal education, often a middle-class background with economic security), there are still many differences across countries and cultures, as Henrich, Heine, & Norenzayan have demonstrated in their seminal 2010 *Behavioral and Brain Science* paper "The WEIRDest people in the world". The acronym reads Western Educated, Industrialized, Rich, and Democratic. These authors demonstrated in an impressive empirical analysis of existing cross-cultural research that the Western Educated, Industrialized, Rich and Democratic people differed in all domains of psychology from the rest of the available worldwide samples. However, it is important to stress that the "rest" is not a homogeneous group, as has often been falsely assumed ("us and the rest").

The rest is a highly diverse crowd, yet all the members of this crowd are different from WEIRD people. This implies that WEIRD people are a very special group, which, moreover, is very small. Estimations vary between 5% and 10% of the world population. In mainstream psychology and its statistical standards, those small numbers of deviating participants would be treated as outliers. Outliers "mess up" the data distributions and, due to their small numbers, they are omitted from samples as irrelevant. Interestingly, in mainstream psychology, the line of argumentation is reversed, and the outliers are declared to be the norm and all other people – the vast majority – to be deviant and, moreover, deficient. This is in itself weird, so that Henrich et al. (2010) conclude: "The findings suggest that members of WEIRD societies, including young children, are among the least representative populations one could find for generalizing about humans" (p. 61).

John Berry (2022) therefore claims that publications in cross-cultural and intercultural psychology should make room for contextual information, going well beyond the usual naming of a cultural or ethnocultural group. This should include a brief ethnographic account of the group, the specific ecological, cultural, and intercultural features that are theoretically linked to the behavior of interest, and the indigenous meaning of the findings.

Yet the problem also extends to the researchers and scientists. Seye Abimbola (2025), e.g., asks in a profound chapter on these issues, "Who are the 'we' who want to know?"

The world of science seems generally WEIRD. It is a closed society where WEIRD participants are primarily studied by WEIRD researchers (Nielsen et al., 2017), steeped in the academic systems that follow the standards of this context (Sanches de Oliveira & Baggs, 2023) with WEIRD procedures and protocols (Broesch et al., 2022). These problems will be discussed more extensively in later chapters.

Although the acronym WEIRD can be criticized because of its unclear and even biased meaning (e.g., Western is not a fixed geographical location; it depends on where one looks), it is nevertheless kept here because it carries an important surplus meaning, i.e., our knowledge base in psychology rests on a very small atypical part of the world's population (members of the middle class in North America, Western Europe, Australia).

This book deals with developmental science, particularly developmental psychology, with a focus on the early years. Interestingly, developmental psychology seems to be the most Western-centric area of all psychology, as Martha Newson and colleagues (2021) argue. They analyzed APA journals between 2016 and 2020 and found that fewer than 4% of developmental articles drew on participants from Asia, Latin America, or Africa. They suspect one reason is the self-orientation of the WEIRD researchers who might seek mini copies of themselves.

Developmental science is thus addressing mainly the universal child. The universal child is the decontextualized and globalized version of a child that should produce generally applicable research findings, which are then expressed in generic language. DeJesus and colleagues (2019) analyzed a corpus of articles published in major developmental psychology journals and found that 73% of articles included at least one generic statement in titles, highlights, or abstracts.

"The universal child" has become a humanitarian movement, as expressed in the title of a ballad by British singer Annie Lennox released in 2010, emphasizing the shared humanity of all children around the world. The song urges us to recognize the innocence and potential of every child regardless of their circumstances. This is in line with the children's rights movement as embodied in the UN Convention on the Rights of the Child, encompassing civil, political, economic, social, and cultural rights. Yet, what is a good intention is not necessarily a good deed. It is undeniable that children need protection, stimulation, and relational security; the children's rights movement, however, represents the claim to universalize a culturally specific idea of childhood as proliferated through Western social science, itself the product of models of post-Enlightment views on personality. Yet, the universal child is an abstraction; it is not a real child. This is comparable to the universal participant in empirical studies, even the universal patient in health sciences (Singh, 2025). There is no child, no participant, no person, regardless of their circumstances, independent of their context. Context is crucial because it provides the background and surrounding details that shape the meaning, interpretation, and relevance of information, communication, or situations. Without understanding the context, responses or decisions may be incomplete, incorrect, or misleading, as they lack the nuanced perspective needed to fully grasp the intent or significance of the subject at hand. As will be demonstrated in more detail later, it is necessary to question the assumption of universality and all of its explicit and implicit implications on the basis of embracing diversity.

WHAT IS MAINSTREAM PSYCHOLOGY?

Throughout this book, the term mainstream is used to characterize the body of psychological knowledge and practice that is based on Western **middle**-class scientific traditions, emphasizing empirical, quantitative research, focusing on individual behavior, cognition, and emotions using standardized methods. It seeks to produce universal laws of human behavior. It is represented in textbooks and encyclopedias as the default and often serves as a template for evaluating grant proposals and reviews of papers in peer-reviewed journals. With some exceptions, these are the only views taught in universities and other educational settings and transferred into application.

Mainstream psychology can be critiqued as Eurocentric and lacking inclusivity, privileging Western worldviews and neglecting non-WEIRD perspectives often labeled as deficient. Other conceptions and ethnographic research are often devalued as unscientific.

Thus, the urgent question remains with whom is psychology dealing and about whom psychology is reporting when generic statements are made and taken for granted as truth universally? The only thing that is safe to say is that mainstream psychology does not talk about around 95% of the world's population, the "neglected 95%", as Arnett has pointed out already almost 20 years ago (Arnett, 2008, see also Thalmayer et al., 2025; Nielsen et al., 2017).

But it is not that we do not know about the psychology and the psychological development of people belonging to these 95%. Scheidecker and colleagues (2023, p. 1) state that "A large body of research on childhood in the majority world exists, e.g. in anthropology, cultural psychology, indigenous psychology. The underrepresentation of the majority world research in the scientific discourse can't therefore not simply be blamed on scarcity of research".

The exclusion of this body of research must therefore be seen as deliberate. One reason may be its evaluation as largely unscientific because it does not readily fit into a predefined epistemic framework consisting of a set of theories, constructs, and measures that are derived from minority world thinking, mainly representing quantitative, variable-focused methodology (mainstream psychology). It must be deeply ingrained in a complex pattern of ideological presumptions, so that "Even the Rat was White", as Guthrie formulated it in 1976.

More and more voices can be heard that qualify this view as biased, distorted, and representing epistemic violence toward the neglected 95% (e.g., Singh, 2024; Scheidecker et al., 2023; Oppong, 2019). What is needed is going WILD, as Bard et al. (2026) demand. This acronym was coined by Newson et al. in 2021, expressing the importance of viewing psychology as **W**orldwide, studied **I**n situ, situated as **L**ocal, and embracing **D**iversity (WILD: Newson et al., 2021). A plea for such an approach in developmental science (and social sciences in general) with the hope of change is the purpose of this book. However, the question remains as to why things do not change despite all the existing awareness and evidence. Reflecting on this crucial topic will be at the end of this book.

2

THE UNIVERSALITY ASSUMPTION

Abstract

Universality is a core assumption of mainstream psychology. It is rooted in different traditions, particularly Western philosophical schools and Christian essentialism. Biological conceptions and neurological findings also incorporate universalistic views. The assumption of universality is closely connected to the assumption of normativity, which expresses that there is one best expression of psychological phenomena that is valid globally. Variability as an inherent ingredient of life is not questioned for plants and animals, yet it is largely denied for humans. Universality and normativity ignore culture as the engine of human behavior and ideas. However, cultures differ with respect to contextual demands. Therefore, variability and multiplicity are the human conditions rather than universality and normativity.

Much of the mainstream social sciences in general and psychology in particular is based on the assumption of universality. The universality assumption, implying that certain principles, norms, or values, including their development, apply to all people and cultures, stems from various sources. In philosophy, it is rooted in the belief in universal truths or essences applying across different instances. It is often tied to concepts like Platonic realism, which implies that there is a true and ultimate reality. This belief has also been a central tenet in religious and philosophical movements, like Christian Universalism, which posits the salvation of all souls by God. Furthermore, the Enlightenment's focus on individual rights and the recognition of the power of the human spirit provided a foundation for modern universalism. The

DOI: 10.4324/9781003672050-3

United Nations' Universal Declaration of Human Rights, which asserts that all human beings are born free and equal in dignity and rights, reflects the assumption of universality in human rights. However, as will be outlined later, as applaudable as this assumption sounds, it nevertheless rests on hidden presumptions that are based on inequality.

Also, biological roots are often claimed as justification for universality, mainly connected to evolutionary theory. Attachment theory is a prime example of this line of thinking, which will be discussed later.

More recently, cognitive neuroscience is promoting the universality assumptions by suggesting that fundamental cognitive mechanisms are shared by all neurologically intact individuals. This is grounded in the study of brain damage in individuals with varying cognitive deficits that led to inferences about the underlying cognitive architecture, assuming a degree of universality in these systems. Kroupin, Davis, and Henrich (2025) even argue that Cognitive Science is a study of human universals. They refer to it as the Newtonian principle, which explicitly or implicitly pervades the theory and methods of most cognitive research. "This is despite at least half a century of sustained critique by cross-cultural and anthropologically oriented researchers and glaring counterexamples..." (abstract). These authors identify the problem as being that only findings that generalize to all humans are regarded as legitimate, an a priori assumption that is ideological, promoting confirmatory research. This problem pertains not only to cognitive neuroscience, but also to many other domains in psychology and social sciences in general. This attitude also reigns in the applied field. For example, Abimbola (2024, 2025) has convincingly demonstrated, intervention studies (in his case, a birth intervention study by Semrau et al. (2020) in Uttar Pradesh) are reinterpreted to confirm previous knowledge. Moreover, poor results, i.e., results not confirming the effectiveness of the intervention, are attributed to context and complexity, which should have been considered beforehand when planning and designing the study. As Abimbola (2025, p. 240) puts it with reference to Semrau et al. (2020):

> The question to ask the authors about unawareness then is: what stopped them from fully reckoning with context and complexity a priori? What stopped them from engaging fully with context and complexity in designing their intervention or in their choice of intervention? Given how much information was available to them from the start, can they claim to be unaware of context and complexity a priori?

The prevailing universalist camp emphasizing common human biological and psychological features is confronted by cultural/cross-cultural scholars emphasizing the importance of context and, relatedly, cultural variation (see, e.g., Cole, 1996; Rogoff & Chavajay, 1995, for historical overviews). These dynamics are central to this book, resulting in a proposal for reconciliation.

The assumption of universality is interrelated with the assumption of normativity, i.e., there is one best way that applies to all. There may be, and obviously are, variations. However, these are being considered as deviations that constitute deficits. The appeasement of those assumed deficits is the motor of tremendous activities in the applied fields, e.g., parenting interventions (see later). The unquestioned but highly problematic scientific and ethical nature of these assumptions is usually not seriously tackled.

What is interesting is that there is generally no questioning about the importance of genetic variability. Everybody accepts that genetic variability is necessary to maintain the existence of humankind and healthy functioning. There is a widespread incest taboo regulating reproduction and genetic relatedness to not jeopardize genetic variability (for a serious discussion, see Bischof, 1985). However, when it comes to the psychological makeup of humans, variability is often denied and universality is postulated. This will be exemplified in more detail later with the case of attachment theory. How can the unquestioned necessary genetic variability go along with psychological uniformity and universality? Wouldn't that imply that the environment, the context of development, does not play a role and that intervention programs and other efforts toward behavioral change would be in vain? In biology, on the other hand, it is unquestioned that plants grow differently in different environments by adapting their structures, functions, and life cycles to suit the specific conditions of their habitat – such as temperature, moisture, light, soil, and altitude. These adaptations help them survive, reproduce, and compete in varied ecological niches. The same principle applies to animals. Why should this principle not apply to humans?

The central but neglected dimension here is culture. Humans live, express, and create culture. Psychological dimensions and functions and their development are embodied in dynamic cultural scripts that operate within genetic frameworks. Therefore, culture and cultural differences must be central to any discussion of human functioning and development. Besides the dominance of WEIRD psychology, there are some cross-cultural studies in several areas of psychology, e.g., compiled in Henrich, Heine, and Norenzayan (2010). The number of such studies has even increased over the last few years. Yet as long as mainly WEIRD researchers study diverse populations with the repertoire of methods developed for WEIRD participants, the gain of knowledge is low. On the contrary, the deficit orientation is reinforced, since WEIRD participants usually get along with WEIRD methodology better than others. It is not the question "how well they can do our tricks", but we should be interested in "how well can they do their tricks", as Mallory Wober stated already in 1972.

In order to understand who "we", "us", and "them" are, we need to deal with the conceptions of context and culture. Both conceptions will be introduced in more detail in the next chapters.

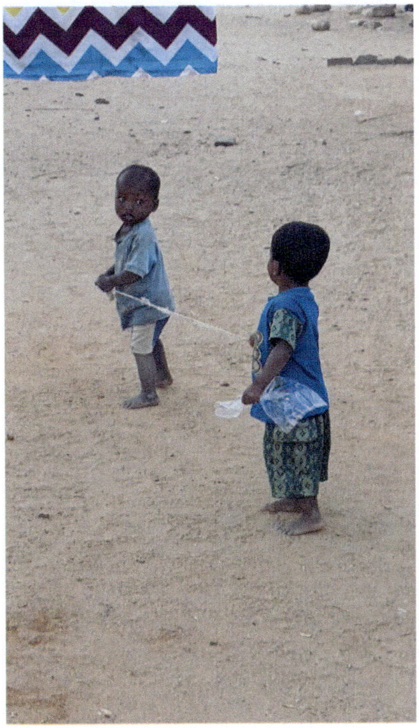

FIGURE 3 Children in Menamaty, southern Madagascar. Copyright Gabriel Scheidecker

3

THE CONCEPT OF CONTEXT

Abstract

The importance of context for behavioral expressions has been elaborated in different approaches over time. Three prominent examples are briefly introduced: Kurt Lewin's field theory, Barker and Wright's behavior setting approach, and Bronfenbrenner's ecological systems theory. Despite the prominence of these approaches, there is hardly a systematic body of research derived from these conceptions. A more recent example with a particular impact in the applied field is Roer-Strier's and Nadan's context-informed perspective. They primarily address risk factors for children's development on these premises.

Especially in cultural/cross-cultural studies, context and culture are closely interconnected. Again, three prominent examples are briefly reviewed: the ecocultural framework by John Berry, the Whiting eco-cultural model, and the developmental niche approach by Super and Harkness. Taking culture into account necessitates the recognition of the contextual affordances and restrictions.

As has been outlined before, context is crucial in understanding the meaning and relevance of behavior and information in general. Although mainstream psychology seems to marginalize context as far as possible (e.g., through standardization of experimental conditions irrespective of environment and participants), there were nevertheless important approaches with different conceptual orientations over historical time to situate behavior into its social and non-social environment. Unfortunately, the understanding of the

DOI: 10.4324/9781003672050-4

contextual embeddedness of psychological phenomena has not conquered psychology as a whole. A few important approaches will be mentioned here, emanating from different historical epochs.

A prominent early example is Kurt Lewin's field theory (Lewin, 1935). The field is thought of as a space in which forces act, as in a gravitational or magnetic field. The field refers to the *total set of interacting forces* (psychological, social, physical) that influence behavior at a given time and not just to isolated stimuli or traits. It takes into account the *dynamic and constantly changing nature* of human behavior. Lewin captured the essence of his approach in the famous formula [$B = f(P, E)$], which defines behavior (B) as a function of the person (P) and the environment (E).

Lewin was closely associated with the Berlin School of Gestalt Psychology and influenced by Gestalt psychologists such as Max Wertheimer, Wolfgang Köhler, and Kurt Koffka. Gestalt psychology emphasizes that *the whole is more than the sum of its parts* and that *perception and experience are organized wholes.*

Lewin's conception has had some impact and has been further developed by some scholars, as discussed by Berry (2022). The cross-cultural psychologist Michael Bond (2013), e.g., has developed a model to account for individual social behavior based on Lewin's formula. He considers that two components of the field are particularly relevant in a person's environment: the "affordances" that permit and support a behavior, and the "normative pressure" to engage in a behavior. These two components provide the "strength" of a situation for the enactment of a particular behavior (see Berry, 2018). Nevertheless, the consideration of the environment as a whole with multiple forces acting at the same time is not reflected in most of the research referring to his approach.

Another general example is the behavior setting approach, developed by Roger Barker (1965; Heft, 2001). He introduced this concept in the 1940s and 1950s as part of his work in *ecological psychology* as an independent branch of psychology (Barker & Wright, 1955). It focuses on how specific settings, including the physical, social, and temporal environment, like a classroom, a church service, or a park, influence and shape the behaviors that occur within them. Essentially, it suggests that the setting itself plays a significant role in determining what people do and how they act.

Behavior setting theory posits that a behavior setting is a combination of a physical environment and a pattern of behavior that regularly occurs within it. The settings are seen as stable, recurring units of human behavior in situ. Gaining some prominence during the 1980s, also in other fields, e.g., pedagogics (see, e.g., Görlitz et al., 1998), the approach has been largely replaced by a contemporary definition of environmental psychology, which addresses questions such as how environments (e.g., noise, crowding, and air quality) affect human behavior and well-being; how humans perceive and interact with their surroundings, e.g., personal space, privacy and environmental attitudes; and how pro-environmental behavior, such as factors that promote sustainable behaviors like recycling, energy saving, or using public transportation can be promoted.

The most prominent example today is certainly Urie Bronfenbrenner's Ecological Systems Theory (1979), which specifically addresses children's development. It proposes that a child's development is influenced by multiple, interconnected environmental systems: the microsystem, mesosystem, exosystem, macrosystem, and chronosystem. These systems are thought of as layers, ranging from the immediate surroundings to broader societal contexts. They interact dynamically to shape an individual's development and behavior.

Reference is mainly made to this early formulation, ignoring that the theory evolved into the more sophisticated Bioecological Model, emphasizing that ongoing, complex interactions between individuals and their environments (proximal processes) are the main drivers of development (Bronfenbrenner & Evans, 2000). Bronfenbrenner criticized the artificial nature of much of the psychological research at the time, particularly lab-based studies with children: "It can be said that much of developmental psychology is the science of the strange behavior of children in strange situations with strange adults for the briefest possible periods of time" (Bronfenbrenner, 1977, p. 513).

This quote criticizes the mainstream methodology, in which many studies are conducted in *lab settings* rather than real-life contexts, children are observed in *unfamiliar environments rather than their familiar environments,* they interact with *strangers* (researchers, not caregivers or teachers), and the *time frame* of studies is usually very short – offering only a *snapshot* of behavior. As a result, these studies often failed to reflect how children really behave and develop in their natural habitat. Although Bronfenbrenner's model is still very popular today and highly referenced, it is often simplified and rarely serves in total as the framework for research designs. It seems that the acknowledgement of the importance of the context is sufficient to go back to normal, meaning laboratory-based, variable-oriented designs that are largely decontextualized.

Based in the field of social work, Dorit Roer-Strier and Yochay Nadan (2020) emphasize context-informed perspectives to study risk, maltreatment, well-being, and protection of children in diverse communities and to develop prevention and intervention programs on these grounds. They adopt a broad conception of context as a matrix of diverse dimensions like culture, religion, class, race, gender, nationality, socio-political context, and more that intersect and influence each other. Contexts influence the construction of meanings of different events and experiences in the lives of individuals and families. Contexts are not fixed and static; they depend on place and time and are therefore subject to change. The approach assumes complexity and hybridity and takes into account power relations between the individual, the family, and the different systems that influence their lives (Nadan & Roer-Strier, 2020).

All of these approaches are important contributions to the understanding of behavior and development in context. They all have in common a holistic view of the dynamics of human functioning and embody the dynamic nature of the person–environment interaction. They differ with respect to the particular focus. Lewin focuses on the person as exposed to field forces with which he/she interacts. Barker and Wright focus on particular contextual units that drive similar behaviors. Bronfenbrenner centers on the individual child as nested in different contexts. Roer-Strier and Nadan are particularly interested in understanding the psychological reality of minorities and the clashes with mainstream views for children's well-being.

It is hard to understand why mainstream psychology is still focusing on a quantitative, variable-oriented, compartmentalized, often deterministic, decontextualized understanding of humans and their development despite the strong arguments for the necessity of a holistic and dynamic perspective. This will be addressed in more detail later.

Except for Roer-Strier and Nadan, who are interested in group-specific views, e.g., Ultra Orthodox Jews in Israel or Ethiopian Jewish migrants in Israel, the focus of these approaches is on general patterns. Culture is not particularly addressed. However, in some branches of cultural and cross-cultural research, the alliance of context with culture was recognized. In these approaches, culture is conceived of as the representation of the environmental parameters of the context in defining norms, values, beliefs, as well as action patterns that are favorable in this context. Moscovici (2000) argues that social/cultural representations are dynamic constructs that emerge from group activities and that integrate external information and group discourses. They represent values, beliefs, and practices that provide individuals with orientation for acting in the world and towards others.

A general example from cross-cultural psychology is John Berry's (2018) eco-cultural model emphasizing how ecological and sociopolitical contexts influence human behavior and psychological diversity. Berry proposes that individuals and groups adapt to their environments through a combination of cultural and psychological processes, considering both individual and collective responses. This framework helps in understanding how people adjust to different cultural settings, particularly in intercultural encounters, such as acculturation processes.

The context-culture combination often emerges out of the collaboration of psychologists with anthropologists. A prominent example is the Whiting ecocultural model (B. B. Whiting, 1980; Whiting & Whiting, 1975). This model links environmental parameters with lifespan development. It starts with the descriptors of the physical environment, like climate and terrain and population density, which interact with the history of humans living in that physical environment. Particular economic and social systems develop, which define children's learning environment, which eventually shapes adult psychology and behavior.

Although genuinely in line with the *zeitgeist* of cultural psychology and anthropology at the time, the Whiting did not deal with biology more than they deemed it necessary. As such, the biological foundation of behavior and development is not particularly emphasized in their writings, mainly confined to fixed genetic programs and hormonal bases of behavior. Although "panhuman biological predispositions" are acknowledged in the sense that "a few prepared or predisposed behaviors ... are learned easily and extinguished only with difficulty" (Whiting & Edwards, 1988, p. 6), the general assumption is that many other kinds of behaviors do not have a prepared basis and most learning "is best described by traditional (social learning) explanations".

However, there is some inconsistency in the writings with respect to the role of the biological foundation of behavior. Whiting and Edwards (1988) refer to "... sensory and receptive equipment and associative predispositions with a long evolutionary history" (p. 6). This statement comes close to the assumption of open genetic programs in evolutionary theory (Mayr, 1988) that bias our learning through "informed hypotheses" or "epigenetic rules" (see Keller, 2007; Keller, 2022a). Thus, one can conclude that the Whiting approach also includes the view that the foundation of learning is evolutionarily prepared (cf. Keller, 2000). Central to both conceptions is the view of development as a response to contextual demands. That is, the starting point for developmental processes in both conceptions is the ecology of the environment (for a differentiated discussion of similarities and differences of both approaches, see Keller, 2004).

The Whiting Ecocultural Model is directly derived from and conceptually underpins the *Six Cultures Study of Socialization*, a landmark cross-cultural research project in developmental psychology and anthropology. It was conducted in the 1950s–1960s and led by *John Whiting* and *Beatrice Whiting* at Harvard University and aimed at observing child-rearing practices and children's learning environments across different cultural groups, representing different ecologies: the rural agricultural Gusii in Kenya, the urban traditional Rajputs in India, the Taira island fishing villagers in Okinawa, Japan, the mountain farming community of the Tarong in the Philippines, the Mixtecans, a traditional agricultural town in Mexico, and Orchard Town, a pseudonym for a small town in New England, USA.

Pairs of researchers, each consisting of an anthropologist and a psychologist, stayed with the communities and studied children's everyday activities, adult-child interactions, peer relationships, discipline and learning, gender roles and expectations, and the roles of mothers, fathers, and siblings in child development in the respective eco-sociocultural realities.

The studies revealed a wealth of insights into the dynamics of the contextual/cultural embeddedness of child development, demonstrating that the way children are raised – what they are expected to do, how they are disciplined, and who teaches them – is deeply rooted in cultural norms. This study was one of the first large-scale, comparative field studies in the field. It contributed to challenging the idea that American/Western (middle-class) child-rearing practices were universal, an idea that earlier anthropologists like Margaret Mead (1954) had already challenged.

Another example is Charles Super and Sara Harkness' (1996) developmental niche approach. The *Developmental Niche* is a conceptual framework that describes how a child's development is shaped by culture-specific settings and practices. It builds on and extends ecological models like Bronfenbrenner's, but with a strong emphasis on cultural meaning systems. A developmental niche consists of three components: the physical and social settings of daily life, i.e., where and with whom the child lives (e.g., household composition, housing, school, and extended family); the customs and practices of child care in terms of daily routines, discipline methods, feeding, sleeping, and schooling – culturally typical practices that structure the child's experience; and the psychology of the caretaker, parental ethnotheories, i.e., caregivers' beliefs, values, and expectations about child development (e.g., independence, obedience, emotional expression, and milestones). This framework highlights how these elements work together to create a unique environment that influences a child's growth and development.

Our own approach of linking context to culture is rooted in these traditions with combining the ecosocial context and evolutionary perspectives (Berry, Whiting & Whiting) with the representational dimension of cultural models (Super & Harkness), framing children's development through evolutionary assumptions of adaptation. We define context in a condensed operationalization of the approaches presented before as a particular pattern of sociodemographic parameters. Especially the level of formal schooling, age at first birth, number of children, and household composition have been demonstrated to be interrelated systematically, representing particular milieus. In our research program, we could differentiate three models, WEIRD, rural traditional, and urban non-WEIRD, which are exemplified with essays about children's learning contexts in a later chapter.

4

THE CONCEPTION OF CULTURE

Abstract

Culture is one of these taken-for-granted meaning systems that, in fact, is used in a wide variety of definitions, and even more often without a definition at all. In the no-definition case, it is equated with a country, society, or any other global group. We follow the cultural psychological/ anthropological tradition of defining culture as shared ideas, beliefs, and norms at the representational level and shared behaviors at the actional level of a group of people living in similar contexts in terms of their life circumstances. Thus, culture is inextricably intertwined with context and can be understood as a representation of context. All humans embody culture inside and outside, yet it is not the same culture. Based on our own and others' research, we differentiate three cultural models: Western middle-class, traditional farmers, and non-Western middle-class according to their sociodemographic profiles.

Culture is a fuzzy and multifaceted term. This is already obvious in different discourse traditions. In the public discourse and the educational practice, culture is mainly understood as art, music, painting, dance, theater, etc., i.e., artistic products and activities.

However, culture is a pervasive construct. Taras and Steel reported in 2009 that a Google search for "cultural" provides over half a billion hits; the Yahoo! search engine even generates a figure of over 2 billion hits. Restricted to academia, the major social science electronic databases provide links to 100,000–700,000 articles.

DOI: 10.4324/9781003672050-5

Sewell (2023) outlined two conceptual approaches. One is culture as a theoretically defined abstract category that can be contrasted with other categories like economy, politics, and biology. The second approach refers to a bounded world of beliefs and practices that is understood as isomorphic with identifiable social groups. It is the second approach that is discussed here. Nevertheless, for this approach, an abundance of definitions can be found in the literature. Already in 1952, Kroeber & Kluckhohn compiled 164 definitions of culture (see also Jahoda, 2012; Kline et al., 2018; Mistry et al., 2013). Although many different aspects are highlighted in these definitions, shared ideas, beliefs, and attitudes (representations) and shared behaviors (actions) of groups of people can be derived as the common denominators of culture (Greenfield & Keller, 2004; Keller, 2019).

It is interesting that the definition of culture is mostly neglected in research activities and publications of the members of the leading society, the "International Association for Cross Cultural Psychology" (see papers in the Journal of Cross Cultural Psychology). Two former presidents, Ype Poortinga and Bill Gabrenya, recently wondered what IACCP members' understanding of culture would be and started a survey: "The concept "culture" is central to our and other academic disciplines, but it is not clear what we are communicating when we refer to the "culture" of a region, nation, or community" (email to the IACCP listserv, February 4, 2026).

Countries cannot be equivalent to culture, since countries are not defined by shared representations and shared behaviors of groups of sociodemographically similar people. Countries obviously host diverse groups with diverse cultures (see also Sanches de Oliveira & Baggs, 2023; and discussion in Taras and Steel (2009) questioning geographic boundaries as optimal for clustering cultures). Culture therefore necessarily embraces diversity. Humans generally acquire, express, and transmit culture, yet it is not the same culture across ecosocial contexts.

Psychology is genuinely cultural (Miller, 1999). Several approaches that deal with culture in psychology have been differentiated, such as cross-cultural psychology (comparing different cultures with respect to behaviors and/or representations), cultural psychology (analyzing the cultural nature of behaviors and representations mainly within one culture), indigenous psychology (studying the psychology of non-WEIRD cultures from a within-culture approach with methods derived from indigenous cultural conceptions), and decolonial psychology (a framework that rethinks psychology through the lens of colonial history, aiming to center the knowledge, voices, and experiences of marginalized, indigenous, and formerly colonized peoples), which incorporate different conceptual ideologies and methodological approaches (e.g., Triandis, 2007; Greenfield & Keller, 2004; Leung, 2012; Bhatia et al., 2025).

Yet there is also substantial variability within these approaches as they overlap, depending on the overall perspective. Therefore, we do not subscribe to any single of these approaches.

As outlined before, the conception followed in this book rests on the eco/psychocultural models briefly presented in the last paragraph (Keller, 2022a).

The reformulation that we have proposed (Keller & Kärtner, 2013) also starts with the environmental conditions, i.e., the context. However, the context is defined more specifically in relation to existing research about child development as the combination of the level of formal education, the age at first birth, the number of children, and the household composition. These dimensions have been empirically identified to form cultural milieus with distinct characteristics (e.g., Keller, 2022a; Lavelli et al., 2019). The milieus follow the Gestalt psychologists' credo that the whole is more than the sum of its parts. Therefore, it does not make sense to control the dimensions of these milieus individually through statistical methods, as mainstream psychology suggests, since their combination carries a different meaning than the pure combination of the individual dimensions. For example, a higher degree of formal education is associated with a later age at first birth, a lower number of children, and a nuclear household structure, which represents a specific learning environment for children's development that cannot be divided into single variables. Singling out the contributions of individual variables statistically would represent an artificial situation that does not match reality. Culture as sharing representations and actions is based on these cultural milieus.

It is important to stress that this is not a static model but one that changes continuously in line with diverse environmental dynamics. For example, it has been documented with national German statistics that the level of formal education is increasing over time, as is the age at first birth, whereas the number of children decreases (Keller, 2017). It is also important to stress that culture is not independent of nurture in accounting for developmental change. In line with Bard, Keller, and Leavens (2026), an epigenetic position is adopted, expressing that

> there is no interaction between nature and nurture because the two are not separate in the first place – rather, what is natural is precisely that organisms develop differently due to their different histories, including the social and environmental aspects of that history.
>
> *(Sanches de Oliveira & Baggs, 2023, p. 22, speaking about Developmental Systems Theory)*

Packer (2026, p. 77) argues that, nevertheless it "....is still popular to think of biology and culture as though they are two completely separate sources of human capabilities", and that "this partitioning of nature and nurture was called into question and, in its place, interactionism became popular". For example, Anne Anastasi wrote that we should no longer assume that "hereditary and environmental factors combine in an additive fashion, ... a more tenable hypothesis is that of interaction" (Anastasi, 1958, p. 197; Packer, 2026, p. 77). However, interaction implicitly assumes two separate entities. Therefore, Evelyn Fox Keller (2010, p. 6) suggests that it is a "mirage" to think that we can distinguish between nature and nurture. As the evolutionary philosopher Eckart Voland (1993) has expressed it: everything is 100% biological and 100% cultural.

With respect to the representational framework of children's development, culture is expressed in cultural models, defining norms, values, beliefs, actions, and action tendencies. Autonomy and relatedness are central dimensions in these cultural models since they represent basic human needs that are defined differently in different environmental milieus and thus represent different cultural models. The cultural models shape child development by defining particular socialization or learning environments, including socialization or developmental goals, parenting ethnotheories, and behavioral practices.

In our research program, we identified three milieus/contexts associated with three cultural models. One is the WEIRD context with a higher degree of formal education, a later first birth, few children, and nuclear households. In this context, the cultural model of psychological autonomy seems to be prevalent, centering around the psychologically independent and self-contained individual and his/her wishes, intentions, preferences, and choices. Of course, relatedness is also important. The autonomous definition of relatedness indicates that social relations are under the control of an individual agent, governed basically by individual needs and self-interests.

A much more common milieu is represented by rural villagers in non-Western environments who usually have a lower level of formal education, earlier first birth, more children, and live in multigenerational households. Here, the cultural model of hierarchical relatedness seems to be prevalent with a communal orientation, embodying social hierarchies and social responsibilities. Of course, autonomy is also important, but it is not individually reflexive but action-oriented, i.e., action autonomy enabling the individual to contribute to the community.

The third model that we could identify represents urban educated families in the majority world with higher levels of formal education like the WEIRD people, and the other dimensions in between the two contexts described above. This cultural model synthesizes the psychological autonomy and the hierarchical relatedness cultural models in different appearances. Thus, individuals are able to be successful in a competitive (work) environment but maintain their communal orientation in the family. School success, e.g., may not be motivated primarily by the will to achieve individually, but for the sake of the family's reputation.

In any case, it is important to stress that one model is not superior to another, as the common deficit perspective would assume. The models just represent differently contextualized cultural models (e.g., Keller & Kärtner, 2013; Keller, 2022a). They also do not necessarily represent the only possible models, which more research in more cultural communities will possibly document.

Of course, there is also a range of intracultural as well as interindividual variation. In the next chapter, more of this variability will be reported.

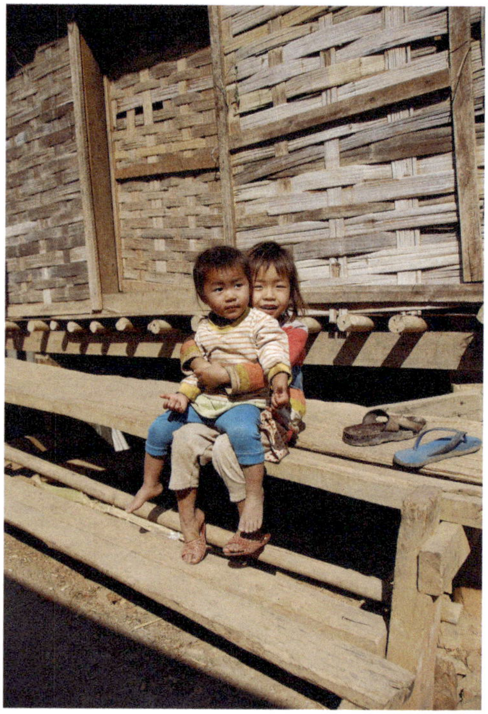

FIGURE 4 Children in a mountain village in Laos. Copyright Kristin Moritz

5

VARIABILITY OF CHILDREN'S LEARNING ENVIRONMENTS

Abstract

Although the amount of research in WEIRD environments by far exceeds the knowledge available from cultural psychological and anthropological studies in other environments, there is nevertheless enough evidence to prove variability as the human condition. Variability concerns household composition and caregiving arrangements. Household composition defines, to a large extent, the caregiving network. Household composition may also change over time, and children may live in different households temporarily or permanently, which has been documented for diverse cultural communities in sub-Saharan Africa. In several cultural communities, children are cared for primarily by other children. As such, they may learn two different interactional scripts at the same time, one with adults and one with other children.

The structure and dynamics of interactional patterns vary across cultural communities, which will be portrayed in fictive portraits of three babies' learning environments.

The previous discussion about the importance of context and culture for behavioral development has advised that the universal and normative assumption of exclusive dyadic interactional patterns does not mirror the reality of children worldwide. The multiple realities of children's learning environments and caregiving arrangements across cultures are documented accordingly by cultural anthropologists and psychologists. There are accounts, e.g., from hunter-gatherer communities like the Congo Basin-based Aka (Hewlett, 1991; Meehan & Hawks, 2013) and Efe (Tronick et al., 1987), pastoralists like the

DOI: 10.4324/9781003672050-6

Fulani in Northwest Cameroon (Yovsi, 2003), or in the South of Madagascar (Scheidecker, 2025), fishermen in Turkey's eastern Black Sea Region (Üskül et al., 2008), informal urban settlements in Kenya (Salinas et al., 2019), and farming villagers like, e.g., the Ivorian Beng (Gottlieb, 2014), the Nigerian Hausa (Marvin et al., 1977), the Kongo-based Aka and Ngandu (Hewlett et al., 1998), the Zaire-based Lese (Morelli, 1987), the Cameroonian Nso, and Indian Gujarati farmers (Abels et al., 2005; Keller, 2022a). Farmer families are studied more than all other groups. That may be due to the fact that they have stable settlements and thus are easier to spot and reach.

The social reality of babies in agrarian communities consists of large intergenerational households. In Nso farming villages in the Bui Division of Northwest Cameroon, households are structured in compounds with a few clay structures roofed with straw or tin. Central to daily life is an open space in the middle of the buildings, in which all household members pursue their daily activities. Children and adults share the same place and the same objects, yet there are social boundaries between the generations (Ndzenyuiy & Keller, 2025).

There is, however, substantial variability in the composition of households and their infrastructure within and across cultural groups. Sophia Becke (e.g., Becke & Bongard, 2018) studied relational patterns of middle childhood in the Nseh Clan in Northwest Cameroon, a cultural group residing next to the Nso. Like the Nso, the Nseh live in compounds. She identified the hearth family as a substructure of the compound family. A hearth family includes the people of the compound who share the same kitchen/hearth. This group spends most of its mornings and evenings together while commonly preparing and sharing food.

Co-residence has been demonstrated to go along with higher accessibility and willingness to participate in taking care of children (Chen et al., 2011; De Villiers, 2011, Schmidt et al., 2023a). Compounds and multigenerational households provide multiple potential caregivers. A broad distinction can be made between caregiving arrangements with functional specialization, where certain caregivers assume only certain responsibilities, and non-specialization, where all caregivers share all responsibilities and act interchangeably (Keller & Chaudhary, 2017).

Household composition may vary temporally. In our research on the Nso culture, we visited families every year but were never sure whom we would meet in the compound. Changes in household composition also mostly imply changes in children's social networks. There is quite some evidence showing that changes in children's care networks, including temporally limited foster care, are common in many societies and considered normative (e.g., Isiugo-Abanihe, 1985; Leinaweaver, 2014). Households are regarded as permeable and fluid, in contrast to the concept of a stable household/family in Western nuclear families.

For example, it is common practice in Baatombu villages in Benin that a child is sent to live with extended family members after the birth of a younger sibling. Children moving in with alloparents help to strengthen mutual-help networks, which are believed to provide a better education. This assumption is so common that among more than 150 older people interviewed, only two had stayed with their biological parents during their entire childhood (Alber, 2004). Similarly, in Batouri, East Cameroon, children are not considered to belong to the parents, but rights to claim children are constantly negotiated, namely, the right to adopt a child from extended family members for company or support with household chores. It is especially common between sisters and brothers to exchange children (Notermans, 2004). Fonseca (2004) describes how children in an urban working-class population in Brazil circulate between different households of extended family members, neighbors, and older siblings, staying for weeks, years, or sometimes forever, and often deciding themselves where they want to live. Similarly, high rates of informal foster care have been reported from rural Ecuador (Walmsley, 2008), black communities in the United States (Miller, 1998), and across several cultural contexts in Oceania (Brady, 2019).

Around one-third of the children in the 30 families in the Lamm et al. (2023) study changed households during the first three years of life, usually coinciding with weaning at around two years. There were no family characteristics that could be generally linked to whether a child changed households or not. Foster care is part of the Nso ideal of collective childrearing (Verhoef, 2005), which ensures children's success and leads to close ties within family networks, similar to childcare arrangements in other African contexts (Alber, 2004; Isiugo-Abanihe, 1985; Leinaweaver, 2014; Notermans, 2004). Whereas older children (starting from six years on) in many sub-Saharan communities are sent to foster parents for education purposes, younger children are fostered by close maternal relatives who nurture them (Bledsoe & Isiugo-Abanihe, 1989). Accordingly, all but one child of the changers in the Lamm et al. sample changed to the grandparents' household and, in one case, to the maternal grandaunt's household. According to Verhoef's (2005) description of Nso foster care arrangements for five- to-eight-year-old children, the household changes in our study could reflect joint ventures. Parents and foster parents were reported to have close relationships and collaborate in childcare. Children were sent to the foster parents for necessary organizational reasons (e.g., a new pregnancy, job seeking). Sometimes the household change was described as a natural development because the grandparents took care of the child during the day anyway, so that the child started to stay overnight. In one case, it was the decision of the child himself. Children deciding about foster care arrangements is a highly interesting aspect of the care arrangements and was also reported in previous studies (Fonseca, 2004; Leinaweaver, 2014; Verhoef, 2005). Nso farmers have been described as a hierarchical community where children learn early to fulfill responsibilities with few opportunities for individual decisions (Keller, 2007; Nsamenang, 1992). However, small children can decide where they want to live, which would be regarded as challenging parental authority in the WEIRD world to the degree that state authorities would be involved. Thus, general conclusions about practices here and there often blur the multifaceted reality.

The duration of the foster arrangements varied greatly, with some children changing back to the original household, others staying in the new household, and most of the children changing back and forth, practically living in both households.

Jessica Leinaweaver (2014) argues that foster care is beneficial when it expands the pool of caregivers rather than replacing one caregiver with another, which allows children to have positive learning opportunities or grants children some autonomy in choosing their place of residence.

There may also be backdrops of these practices, as e.g., Waris Dirie has documented in her book "Desert flower" (Dieri, 1999). Like many children from rural sub-Saharan villages, Waris was sent to urban relatives. Her father arranged her trip to London to work in the household of the Somalian ambassador to Great Britain, who was her uncle. As an unpaid maid in the Somalian embassy, she never saw a school from inside, although she was only 13 or 14 years old when she arrived in Great Britain.

There are different numbers of caregivers for a baby in different locations reported in the literature. Tronick, Morelli, and Ivey (1992) analyzed the social networks of small Efe children. They demonstrated that one to four different children were observed in regular social contact with five-month-olds, and that one to six different children with three-year-olds within a typical hour. At the same time, five-month-olds were likely to come into contact with up to four adults, three-year-olds with two to seven adults. However, there are more people around providing ambient social stimulation.

In the Nso community, the mother plays an important role in being the most prevalent caregiver during the first three years of life within a network of caregivers. The frequent involvement of mothers is mainly based on breastfeeding. Nso women usually wean their infants in the third year (Yovsi, 2003; Yovsi & Keller, 2007). During the first few months, infants are exclusively breastfed, and mothers are mostly available for breastfeeding on demand. Lamm et al. (2023) report that in their study, however, only one child was reported to favor the mother over other caregivers, indicating that presence and preference are not identical. Also, the mother's involvement changes substantially, with the most dramatic decrease toward the end of the first year. The decline of maternal involvement is related to the reduction of breastfeeding as infants start taking solid foods. Once complementary feeding has been introduced, infants can be cared for by other caregivers for longer periods of time, so that alloparental involvement increases. These findings further strengthen the argument that the mother is one among many and not necessarily the most important caregiver (Keller & Chaudhary, 2017).

The Nso pattern of alloparenting is similar to the Madagascan example, where mothers also represent major caregivers during the first two to three years (Scheidecker, 2025). Also, Madagascan Menamaty mothers almost exclusively provide physical care, while Nso mothers also reported participating in play and other social activities, at least during the first year of life (Lamm et al., 2023). Scheidecker's meticulous ethnographic research has revealed important insights into differences between adult care and children's care. He convincingly demonstrates that children in Menamaty are provided with two parallel socio-emotional developmental scripts: a hierarchical-relational script and an egalitarian-autonomous script (Scheidecker, 2025; Scheidecker, 2023). Based on his findings and other studies, he argues that: (1) interactions with caregivers and similarly aged children are distinct and complementary, fulfilling different but equally important needs; (2) children experience and acquire both socio-emotional modes simultaneously from the first year onward rather than sequentially; (3) the egalitarian developmental script exists independently of the hierarchical script rather than as an extension; and (4) that bonds between children are deeper and have more dimensions than what is normally implied by the terms "peers" or "friendships" (Scheidecker, 2025). With adult caregivers, children experienced the fulfillment of bodily needs and physical security, while with other children they explored their surroundings and engaged in cognitively stimulating interactions. Emotionally, relationships with adult caregivers were characterized by calmness and the regulation of negative emotions, whereas relationships with other children were emotionally stimulating, allowing for the experience and sharing of both intense anger (and other negative emotions) and joy (and other positive emotions). Similar distinctions in activities have been reported for mothers and fathers in WEIRD samples, with mothers being more calming and regulatory and fathers being more stimulating and exciting (e.g., Dagan & Sagi-Schwartz, 2018). The differences are often integrated into a hierarchical system with the mother granted primacy because the regulatory function is considered more important than the stimulatory one. However, the differences in the symmetry of interactions in the Madagascan villages, where interactions with adult caregivers were distinctly asymmetrical and hierarchical while those with similarly aged children were symmetrical and egalitarian, are considered equally important.

Scheidecker (2025) concludes that (T)these two socio-emotional pathways…do not emerge in a sequential fashion but instead coexist from the first year of life. This is due to the fact that children in Menamaty receive consistently distinct social and emotional experiences from caregivers and similarly aged peers. These two types of social partners complement each other by offering different, but equally essential, socio-emotional experiences. This challenges prevailing assumptions in developmental science – especially those rooted in attachment theory – that position the caregiver-child relationship as the primary foundation for all subsequent social relationships. The coexistence of those different communication patterns may be prevalent in other rural communities as well, where children's participation in children's social worlds is reported. Scheidecker's groundbreaking research should instigate more systematic studies of children's social worlds. Especially the assumption of equal importance should also be reconsidered within the attachment framework with respect to differences between mothers and fathers. In normative WEIRD families, children also grow into two scripts at the same time, yet they are both provided by adult caregivers and differ in terms of assumed relevance for attachment formation.

Generally, the relational network of these village children is instrumental in priming other parameters of children's learning environment, which may go equally unnoticed and be taken for granted as the implicit assumptions in the WEIRD childcare philosophy.

5.1 Interactional dynamics across cultural communities

The presence of multiple people in the same place facilitates polyadic communication patterns. Polyadic, as different from dyadic, implies that people are involved in different communication threads at the same time and, moreover, witness those in which they do not actively participate. This applies to adults and children equally. The village social environment assigns importance to nonverbal communication, which is secondary in the WEIRD world, where the spoken word counts. The credo of turn-taking, i.e., listening quietly to the speaker until he/she finishes, before one's own verbal communication is delivered, is replaced by co-occurring, overlapping behavior. For example, in some communities in Hawaii, it is regarded as impolite to let somebody finish talking before starting oneself. The overlapping mode already starts in infancy. Maya Gratier (2003) observed that Indian migrant mothers in the USA started talking while their few-month-old babies were still vocalizing, whereas US middle-class mothers waited until the baby ended before reacting. A similar pattern was found comparing Nso farmer mothers with German middle-class mothers (Keller & Otto, 2009). The fast but distinct reaction in WEIRD families (contingent responsiveness) is regarded as an important condition for children developing an early sense of self as separated from others and self-efficacy as the capability to exert control in social situations. The overlapping, co-occurring mode (Saraswathi & Pai, 1997), on the other hand, allows the baby to perceive him/herself as part of a whole, paving the way for the development of a communal identity.

This distinction is pervasive throughout life. For example, the WEIRD social etiquette asks for concentration on one thing at a time, whereas the social etiquette for many rural communities asks for splitting attention. It has been documented in several communities (Keller, 2022a) that visual attention is directed at chores, e.g., preparing meals, sweeping the floor, and the like, whereas bodily attention is with the baby who is lying on the lap, sitting on the hip, or bound to the back. This also stresses the prevalence of bodily, proximal communication, at least between babies/children and adults (see Scheidecker, 2025; Keller & Kärtner, 2013).

Since babies are always in close (bodily) contact with other people, there is no need for security objects. Commercial toys are rarely found in the villages anyway.

In our own research project in the Nso villages, we once brought a big toy doll that the daughter of a German collaborator wanted to send as a gift to the Nso children in the village. For her, it was a precious gift, which was not easy to give away. Yet the Nso children hardly took notice of it and finally placed it somewhere remote in the house. We never saw it again.

This little episode could be a metaphor for many aid programs and interventions, expressing that a good thought is not a good deed. Nevertheless, children everywhere play with objects, which, in the village environment, they often manufacture themselves from available material like grass, wood, and the like. When they have finished playing, they just leave the objects behind, contrary to the importance of individual property in WEIRD philosophy.

Another differential dimension of communicative patterns across cultures is emotional display rules. As has been reported before, positive emotional displays are the default condition in WEIRD communities. In non-WEIRD communities, different social scripts have been described. There are studies that demonstrated emotional neutrality being the favorite facial display. In the Nso rural community, e.g., Otto (2014) demonstrated that a stranger approaching a one-year-old Nso child did not cause an anxious or frightened facial display, and possibly crying, as is usual for WEIRD children. Most of the rural Nso children had a neutral face and demonstrated approach behavior toward the stranger, like stretching their arms. David Lancy (2022) reported in his eminent anthropological documentation that caregivers in non-Western cultures are less emotionally outgoing, especially toward infants and toddlers. For example, emotional engagement like eye contact, expressive talking, or smiling of adults toward children is minimal, e.g., in the Gusii (LeVine et al., 1994), like among the Nso (Keller, 2022a), and in many other rural communities (for more examples see Otto & Keller, 2014; Gottlieb, 2004; Quinn & Mageo, 2013). Scheidecker's analysis adds a new dimension to these findings, demonstrating that emotional neutrality is not the overall communicative pattern, but is specific to the social partners. The Metamaty Madagascan children of his study learn emotional neutrality within hierarchical settings (children with adults) and emotional expressiveness in egalitarian settings (children with children) concurrently. He argues that children in Menamaty thus receive consistently distinct social and emotional input and feedback from caregivers and similarly aged peers (Scheidecker, 2025). Since researchers, including us, transported the bias stemming from their own worldview that mainly adults are caring for children, mainly interactions between children and adults were studied, neglecting the study of peer interactions among younger children.

The complementary pattern does not seem to be unique to the Menamaty context, but also exists in similarly structured communities. Scheidecker reports some indicators in this direction in the anthropological literature (e.g., Leiderman & Leiderman, 1974; LeVine et al., 1994). An important contribution was Thomas Weisner and Ronald Gallimore's (1977) article "My Brother's Keeper", where the prevalence of nonparental caregivers with a specific focus on child caregivers was demonstrated to exist in many places.

Personal observations in the Northwestern Cameroonian Nso community also confirm these differentiations. Whereas Nso children avoid eye contact and facial mimical expressions with adults and only contribute brief verbal statements when asked, they are mimically quite expressive and talkative with peers.

Children growing up in rural non-Western villages obviously experience a complex environment in which they learn to differentiate between contexts and behave according to the respective context. This complexity must have consequences for their emotional and cognitive development (see detailed discussion in Scheidecker, 2025).

Thus, contrary to the beliefs and assumptions about impoverished and deficient environmental input, the rural non-WEIRD children experience abundant social and cognitive stimulation in their natural habitat. In comparison, WEIRD children are rather deprived due to the pervasive ideology of the child that needs protection from stimulation. This seeming contradiction will be discussed later.

Children's learning environments are obviously differently organized, providing different learning opportunities, which necessarily lead to different developmental pathways (Weisner, 2002). In the following sections, three baby stories will be portrayed, exemplifying the three types of learning environments. The babies described are not real but are composed from the results of our cross-cultural research program in these three contexts. Existing studies from cultural psychologists and anthropologists from non-WEIRD farmer communities are also integrated (e.g. Mezzenzana, 2023).

5.1.1 Portrait of a small baby in a WEIRD family from Berlin, Germany

Justin was born to a 36-year-old mother and a 38-year-old father in Charlottenburg, a posh district of Berlin (west), the capital of Germany. His parents first met at the campus of the Free University, when his mother started studying journalism and communication sciences and his father started law school. They sat by chance next to each other in the central introductory event for first-semester students at FU. Full of curiosity about what the new phase in their lives would keep ready for them, they started a conversation about what they were studying, where they were living, and what their impressions of being a new student at FU were. Justin's mother is a native Berlin girl, still living in her parents' apartment in Charlottenburg, but looking for a place in a shared apartment, which she thought was more appropriate for a student life. Yet at the beginning of the semester, finding something suitable is extremely difficult because of high demand. Since she has a safe place in her parents' apartment, she is quite relaxed in her search. Justin's father recently moved to Berlin when he was informed that his application to law school was successful. He lives temporarily in a youth hostel because he did not find a place in a student's home or a shared apartment. However, he is also quite optimistic because he can count on his parents' support.

The two liked each other and started dating. Yet after a couple of months, they both realized that they were not ready to commit to a long-term relationship because their studies and careers had priority at that time. Therefore, they split on good terms.

Unpredictable as life is in their worldview, they met again by chance in a big blue bus running from Santa Monica to Westwood and UCLA. Both had enrolled and were accepted as exchange students at the same time at UCLA.

Familiar with using public transportation from Berlin, they were surprised that bus riding was considered a low-income activity in Los Angeles. Yet, both had maintained their curiosity and wanted to participate in the "real world".

Justin's mother lived as a paying guest with a family in Santa Monica, where she had been an Aupair girl for a year during her high school education. Justin's father lived in a cooperative housing room in Westwood and occasionally went to the seaside in Santa Monica. Their earlier affection for each other was immediately back again, and was perhaps intensified through being expatriates. They grew together over the months, spending a lot of time together when they were not involved in their studies. Eventually they also moved together and started thinking about a joint future in Berlin. They went back and successfully finished their studies with MAs. They found a nice apartment on the fifth floor of a founding area building around Savignyplatz with a lift ending on the fourth floor. Justin's father started his obligatory two-year legal traineeship. Justin's mom started as a freelance journalist specializing in science journalism. Both were fully engaged in their careers but nevertheless enjoyed the spare time they had together, going to nice restaurants, traveling, and visiting museums and art galleries. They enjoyed their independent life but nevertheless started thinking about founding a family.

Justin's mom became pregnant when she was 35 years old. She was very happy when she found out about the pregnancy, as was Justin's dad. She stopped immediately drinking an occasional glass of wine that she had loved to do before. They did all the medical check-ups and, when the first three months had passed, they informed family and friends. Especially their parents were very relieved, since they had developed concerns over the last few years about ever becoming grandparents at all. Justin's mom started reading all kinds of books about children's development, browsing through magazines and looking for a midwife, and checking birth hospitals. Both had never been in touch with a baby before and were quite nervous about what they had to expect. Justin's mom gave birth on time in a hospital they had carefully selected, with Justin's dad being present. The birth was 20 hours long and physically and emotionally draining. They all stayed together another day in a family room in the hospital before they returned to their home. They were both very tense because they had never held a baby in their arms before. They wanted to be the best parents for their baby and do everything right to give Justin a good start in his life. However, life with the baby was quite a challenge for them. Their daily routines were upside down. They couldn't get enough sleep. Justin's mom was on maternity leave for a year and Justin's dad took two months of paternity leave, so that the new family could settle. After those two months, he would return to work full time in the law firm where he was employed. So far, they took turns caring for their son, as far as it was possible, since Justin was breastfed on demand. That should be continued at least for three months, which was the recommendation of the pediatrician. Breastfeeding was going smoothly, and Justin's mom enjoyed looking into Justin's eyes during breastfeeding. She felt that this was a special time for bonding and relationship building because it was their exclusive shared experience. Justin's dad was not jealous of their quality time because he knew his time would be coming when Justin got older, taking him to soccer games or other activities that Justin's mom was not really fond of.

Justin's sleep was irregular and he cried a lot. Justin's mom read about programs and sleep coaching (like "every baby can sleep") but they agreed that they found these methods inappropriate. Instead, Justin's mom tried to find a group of young mothers in the same situation with the help of her midwife, where they could exchange information and support each other. She found a women's group, which was immensely helpful because all the women had the same experiences and talking with like-minded women was a relief. Also, the pediatrician reassured her that this was a transitory period that many families went through, which does not impair future healthy development. Nevertheless, sleeping remained a topic, and Justin's parents found out that body contact was helpful to soothe him. Consequently, more and more often, Justin slept with his parents in their bed. They wouldn't tell anybody, but in some face-to-face encounters with other mothers from the women's group,

Justin's mom found out that other moms did the same. All the women agreed that babies had to be protected from overstimulation, i.e., not exposed to many people, facing mom or dad only, and being in a quiet environment. They also consented that children should have their own world, their own room with child-friendly furniture, child-friendly decoration, and toys.

Justin's mom talked a lot to him in all kinds of situations. She had read that talking to babies is very important because it stimulates their cognitive development. When he was awake, she asked him what he wanted to do, what he did not want to do, what he preferred, what he liked, what is going to happen tomorrow, and how he felt. She was anxious to present him with choices and pretended that he had decided on one option. She constantly praised him for what he was (so strong already), what he did (you're telling me stories), and what he intended (you want to play on your own, big boy).

While talking to him, she tried to maintain as much eye-to-eye contact as possible, as eye-to-eye contact is considered crucial for children's socio-emotional development in the books and guides that she had read. They had large amounts of baby toys, which they had bought, and which family and friends had brought as gifts. She showed him toys and explained them to him to stimulate his interest. During all these interactions, Justin was lying on his back in his crib or on a mat on the floor when his mother bent over him with their faces close together. She touches him occasionally with a fingertip, but there was not much body contact. When he got fussy or cried, she asked him what the reason could be, although he had been fed and diapered shortly before. She was waiting for signals that would help her find out what he had. As the last measure, she took him in her arms and rocked him and moved him rhythmically. Otherwise, she did not support his trials to sit because the pediatrician warned against early sitting because the body would not be mature enough.

Mothers in her group reported more radical ways to deal with crying, like fixing the baby on a washing machine during spinning, driving around in a car, or moving a baby stroller over cobblestones. Sometimes Justin's father took over and walked with him in a baby sling on his body for some early morning hours in their neighborhood so that his mom could get some sleep. As it turned out, some mothers in the women's group were adherent to the attachment parenting approach, devoting a caregiver's (mostly moms') unconditional and exclusive attention to the baby 24/7. Justin's mom basically agreed that babies need full and exclusive attention, but she was not ready to give up her occasional, nevertheless short, meetings with friends and colleagues to keep track of what was going on outside her family. These meetings gave her energy and perspectives. Yet, she had a bad conscience for not being available for Justin during these moments. There is a general agreement that childcare is child-centered, with children being treated as quasi-equal conversational partners from day one on.

5.1.2 Portrait of a small baby in a North West Cameroonian Nso farming family

The Nso are an ethnic group residing in the Northwest of Cameroon. Due to political turmoil, the traditional ruling system with a king (Fon) and a hierarchy of dignitaries living in a strict system of conventional rules and customs has been softened. However, traditional lifestyles are still in place, mixed with more modern elements. Extended, multigenerational patriarchal households are located in compounds. Traditional courtship often begins with community introductions, where families play a key role in connecting potential partners. While traditional methods are still practiced, modern dating practices like meeting through friends, at social events, or online are also becoming more common. In any case, it is expected that one marries within one's own ethnic group. Women usually marry in their late teens and early twenties, with men usually being a couple of years older. Depending on marriage agreements, men can also be substantially older than women. Marriage is mandatory to become recognized by society. Single mothers live stigmatized in their parents' compound.

Junior's parents both grew up in the market town of Kumbo, the capital of the Bui district in North West Cameroon, close to the Nigerian border. His mother is the eldest of eight siblings, growing up in a farming family, cultivating potatoes, beans, maize, cocoyams, manioc, pumpkins, and huckleberry. They sold their products in the local market, with the children taking turns at the market stall. Junior's mom is the only one in the family who received some higher education. She underwent teacher training and teaches in one of the local preschools. His father is the eldest son of nine siblings, growing up in a farming family raising animals like chickens, pigs, goats, and sheep. They also cultivated some vegetables and staples like corn and manioc for their own consumption. Three of the boys got some higher education, with Junior's father receiving training as a kind of vet, mainly vaccinating animals. Junior's mom and dad met after church activities when they hung out for a little while with friends. They never spent time alone, but they both felt drawn to each other. Junior's dad talked to the elderly in his family and asked for permission to marry Junior's mom. This involved his family approaching the family of the bride and settling the marriage negotiations in case they agreed to the marriage.

The marriage was settled and immense preparations started. With 250 guests, it was not really a big wedding, but numerous tasks had to be completed, including dresses in the traditional colors and patterns for the bride and groom and other dresses for the bridesmaids. All the dresses for the bridesmaids looked alike. Looking the same signaled the community spirit, the feeling of togetherness, and communal identity. Incredible amounts of food were prepared; many liters of palm wine, lots of cases of beer, whiskey, and much more had to be organized. Chairs, tables, and tents needed to be rented, and much more. It was a several-day event where, in the end, all were happy.

The young couple moved into a brick house close to Junior's father's home compound. The fact that they could start in their own house is a sign of modernity and also related to their educational status, because both had paid jobs. A couple of younger relatives lived with them, helped with household chores, and worked in the garden where they were growing vegetables and keeping chickens. Junior's mom got pregnant soon and gave birth to Junior when she was 22; his dad was 24. With the birth of their first child, they changed their names to mother of Junior and dad of Junior, which is a long-held tradition. Names are often changed during one's lifetime because identity is not fixed to a single address.

Caring for a baby was natural to Junior's parents, since they had cared for younger siblings, cousins, and neighbor's children since they were two to three years old. Childcare is a common obligation and responsibility with many people participating, including relatives, neighbors, children, adolescents, adults, and elderly people. Both parents continued working after birth, relying on a natural caregiving environment for their firstborn. In fact, he was constantly in close body contact with somebody, being carried on hips and backs and lying on laps. He experienced a lot of body stimulation this way because he was drawn into others' rhythms when they walked and moved. This also resulted in him developing as a part of a social system. "I am because we are" is a sub-Saharan African proverb expressing this ideal of interrelatedness.

Junior was breastfed on demand by his mom, and, when she was not available, also by another lactating neighboring woman. Breastfeeding is crucial because people think that you only become a Nso through breastfeeding.

From birth onward, Junior participated in the real world of his community, sharing the same space and basically also the same activities. Therefore, he was also usually facing out when being held to perceive what was going on around him. Caregivers tended him while doing their chores and usual activities, with co-occurring attention, i.e., their bodily attention was on him, reacting immediately to his body signals, while their visual attention was on their work and activities.

Anthropologist Francesca Mezzenzana (2023) reports from the Runa people, an agrarian community living in Ecuador, about similar learning environments,

> ...Runa children participate fully in adults' lives, overhearing complex conversations between adults on difficult topics, helping with domestic tasks, taking care of their younger siblings. Participating in the adult world means that sometimes children can get frustrated, or denied what

> they want, or feel deeply dependent on others. At the same time, there is so much that they gain: they learn to pay close attention to interactions around them, to develop independence and self-reliance, and to forge relationships with their peers. Most importantly, in this adult world, they are constantly reminded that other people – their parents, their family members, their neighbours, their siblings and peers – also have desires and intentions.

This is pretty much also the philosophy of the Nso farmers and many other traditional farmers in different countries of the Global South.

Junior spends a lot of time with the children living in his house, but also in both sets of grandparental households. All these people include him in their daily activities so that he has a rich environment to observe, to learn, and to pitch in. Junior also spends occasionally a week or two with a paternal aunt and her husband in a village, not too far from Kumbo. In their neighborhood, an elderly widow is living all alone because her children moved to the city. She loves Junior's company and often takes him for hours and indulges him with puff-puff, a local pastry that she prepares for him.[1]

Junior always sleeps with somebody, which implies that he does not have a regular place to sleep or even his own bed. He smoothly transfers from caretaker to caretaker from early on. When he wakes up at night, he feels the warmth of another person and falls asleep again fast. He never cried much, particularly not for longer bouts of time. There was always somebody reacting immediately. When his mother was around, breastfeeding was the normative response. Walking around with Junior on the back and moving rhythmically is often used to anticipate slight body tensions that were perceived through close body contact without layers of clothes between the bodies. Body language with nonverbal regulation was the primary communication mode during the first year. Junior could walk independently at nine months and was toilet trained by seven months.

Generally, all agreed that babies should find their place in their community fast and become responsible members of the community.

5.1.3 Portrait of a Baby in a Middle-Class Family in Delhi, India[2]

Nilay's parents both come from urban middle-class Hindu families living in Delhi. They each hold university degrees – his mother studied Home Science, and his father is a pharmacist. Both had spent a semester abroad: his mother in the UK and his father in Australia. They first met through mutual friends. In urban middle-class circles, especially among those with similar academic or professional backgrounds, social introductions often happen through such networks.

When it became clear that they had serious intentions toward each other, they sought their families' consent. Nilay's maternal family insisted on involving an astrologer to assess the couple's compatibility and to determine an auspicious date for the wedding. Once everything was aligned to everyone's satisfaction, wedding preparations began.

A Hindu marriage is a major event, often requiring several months of preparation. Leading up to the wedding, various rituals were performed, such as the henna (mehendi) ceremony, a musical evening (sangeet), and the turmeric (haldi) ceremony. The wedding itself, attended by 300 guests, took place in a hotel and lasted several days, filled with food, music, and dancing. Among the key rituals was the *pheras*, during which the couple walks around the sacred fire seven times, each round symbolizing a specific vow related to their roles and commitment in married life.

After the wedding, Nilay's mother left her parental home to join her husband's household, in keeping with traditional Hindu practice. Although both families hoped for grandchildren soon, Nilay's parents wanted to travel first. They planned visits to the countries where each of them had studied abroad. Upon returning to Delhi, Nilay's father began working as a pharmacist, while his mother planned to pursue a PhD. Her long-term goal was to start her own business, which she believed would offer her greater flexibility to balance career and family life.

Nilay was born three years after his parents' marriage, when his mother was 26 and his father 28. His mother was his primary caregiver, but many others took active roles in his upbringing – his father, both sets of grandparents, and other members of their extended family, who fortunately lived not too far away. The presence of others to care for the baby was also considered important for the well-being of the mother, who was also thought to be in need of care and nurturance. For this reason, the new mother is usually sent to be in her natal home, with her own parents, for the delivery. Nilay's mother also went to her parents' home for the delivery, surrounded by several family members who were available to assist and advise. The birth itself took place in a nearby maternity hospital. The young mother's own family members ensure her complete comfort, care, and nourishment during this difficult period. Keeping the new mother and child restricted to the hospital and/or home is valued for the first couple of months, especially the first 40 days after birth.

Massage was an important part of Nilay's early life. He received his first massage just a few hours after birth, and it became part of his daily routine throughout much of his first year. A *dai* – an experienced elderly woman from the neighborhood – visited regularly to gently massage him with herbal oils. Massage is believed to strengthen the baby's body and harmonize life energy (*prana*). Facial massage is also thought to promote symmetrical features, which is a commonly held beauty ideal. Nilay's mother would sometimes massage him as well, believing it would help strengthen their bond.

Nilay was breastfed on demand. During breastfeeding, his mother held him close for face-to-face contact, speaking softly to him and cherishing their time together.

Nilay never slept alone. He usually slept near his mother, but occasionally stayed with other relatives or grandparents in their homes. From an early age, he learned to sleep in different places, always with familiar people nearby. For the entire extended family, the idea of a baby sleeping alone – especially in a separate room – was unimaginable. They viewed constant physical closeness as essential to a child's well-being. Alongside, as the baby grew older, it was also believed to be good for him to lie on his own and fuss a little bit before being attended. Crying was believed to strengthen the lungs and general well-being.

During waking hours, Nilay was almost always in physical contact with his mother or another caregiver. He experienced frequent face-to-face interaction, with caregivers talking to him about the world around him. He was also often carried facing outward so that he could observe his environment, and after the first several weeks of restrictions, visitors would visit the family, view and hold the baby, and talk to him to join in the joy of a newborn. From the very beginning, he was surrounded by a safe and supportive social network, from which he gradually learned to participate in shared life.

The first year of a middle-class Hindu baby's life is rich in meaning, love, care, and spiritual practices. Each developmental milestone is celebrated and imbued with ritual significance to support the child's physical, emotional, and spiritual growth.

Soon after birth, Nilay received a small dot of *kajal* between his eyebrows, on the forehead, or even behind one ear, to protect him from the *buri nazar* (evil eye), a common belief in many Indian families. His naming ceremony (*naamkaran*) was held on the 11th day after his birth. The name *Nilay* – which means "abode" or "dwelling" in Sanskrit – was chosen based on astrological charts that recommend the first letter of the name, allowing the family to pick one that they like.

When Nilay was about six months old, a special ritual marked his first taste of solid food. He was fed a ceremonial porridge sweetened with ghee and jaggery. This milestone, known as *annaprashan*, is a significant cultural moment symbolizing the child's growth and transition into a new phase of life.

A couple of months later, another important ceremony, *Mundan*, represented another significant rite of passage in Nilay's life, symbolizing purity. Mundan is a tonsure ritual where a child's head is shaved for the first time. A barber or priest performs the shaving, and the head is often washed with holy water and treated with turmeric and sandalwood paste to soothe and heal. The shaved hair is offered to a deity, symbolizing devotion and gratitude. The ceremony for Nilay was performed in his ninth month because it had to be in an odd-numbered month. It was scheduled based on his horoscope and auspicious astrological conditions.

Generally, besides health and well-being, Nilay's parents, together with their families of origin, wanted to instill moral values, responsibility, and a good sense of self so that Nilay would become a competent and happy person.

5.2 Similarities and differences

The three portraits are prototypes that summarize typical baby and family stories for the three contexts. The portraits embody different socialization/learning environments, demonstrating that children grow up in different cultural realities and scripts. However, it is not all about differences; there are also similarities that we have discussed as structural universals before (Keller, 2022a). The major similarity is that all children grow up in social networks composed of people who take responsibility for their thriving and well-being. To become competent adults in their environments, children all over the globe have to address similar developmental tasks. They all have to learn to walk, to talk, to relate to others, and to develop a sense of self. But children learn to achieve these developmental milestones in different social contexts, with different social partners, at different times, depending on the cultural emphasis on the particular task in the particular environment. This also pertains to the interpatterning of these tasks in developmental pathways. The principle of equifinality (see Cicchetti & Rogosch, 1996; Gernsbacher et al., 2026) expresses that the developmental achievements like talking, relating, etc. may look quite different in their phenotypical appearances. They are embedded in different cultural meaning systems and marked with different rituals and celebrations.

Babies in the different environments experience different emphases on learning daily routines. WEIRD babies are expected to develop regularity soon, i.e., get used to stability in time and place. This refers to sleeping, e.g., developing regular sleeping patterns and getting used to sleeping in the same place. Babies in rural traditional households are expected to flexibly pitch into the activities of their caregivers. They sleep whenever they get tired, wherever they are at that moment. Urban lifestyles generally ask for more regularity, so middle-class families in the Global South also pay more attention to regular rhythms.

Babies in the different environments learn developmental achievements at different times, depending on the cultural emphasis placed on the specific achievement. Based on the ideology of child-centered care, WEIRD babies should develop according to their own pace, at their own tempo. Yet, one of the many contradictions in the WEIRD upbringing and education is that this, in fact, only applies to some developmental domains. For example, it is believed to be a no-go to train motor development; however, mothers tend to compare their babies with others and get concerned when they perceive that other babies are more "advanced", as defined by developmental timetables that their pediatricians have in mind and that are displayed in pediatricians' practices, as well as in day care institutions. Another example is that despite the credo of individual variability, there is a strong belief in a fixed sequence of motor development. Thus, crawling is considered a necessary phase to precede walking to avoid a negative impact on brain development. This is a myth, as longitudinal observations of individual babies' development have revealed (Michaelis, 2006). Yet this myth is maintained until today. The cultural emphasis is on cognitive development and cognitive stimulation to foster brain development, which is supposed to be crucial. Toys, especially so-called educational toys (e.g., blocks, shapes, cut-out pieces, puzzles), are recommended in parent guidebooks (and also in parenting interventions addressed later). The general advice to talk much to the baby should foster language development, because it is believed that language is acquired in dyadic dialogues with directly addressing the baby exclusively (Hart & Risley, 1992; but see Sperry et al., 2018; Gilkerson et al., 2017). Mentalizing, i.e., talking about inner states, assumed desires, wishes, preferences, and intentions of the baby, is believed to foster cognitive development and to contribute to parent-child attachment (Keller, 2022b). These strategies, of course, are also training, but are not recognized as such. They are considered to be stimulation, which is part of quality parenting (see, e.g., the Nurturing Care Framework, discussed later).

In general, the focus is on the inner world, the individuality, and uniqueness of the baby. The caregiver is supposed to transmit to the baby that he or she is an extraordinary and exceptional individual who deserves and can expect all the exclusive attention and care. In several policy statements, such as the Children's Right Charta, issued in 1989 by the UN General Assembly, this is an undisputable right of all children. This socialization strategy and learning environment thus adheres to the cultural model of psychological autonomy/psychological relatedness.

The cultural emphasis in non-WEIRD traditional families is on early motor competence, so that children become independent of others' efforts to carry them around. Early walking is trained, e.g., in the Nso community, by moving the baby up and down, which is supposed to strengthen bodily development and especially the joints (Keller et al., 2002). If a baby does not walk independently toward the end of the first year, special training devices are used, like self-made walkers or two rods at the height of the baby's hands with the baby put inside and strongly encouraged to practice walking. Other children are around to supervise the child, help, and correct if necessary.

Children lying most of the time on their back, as usual in WEIRD environments, are believed to develop serious problems, leading to death in the worst case. On the other hand, German middle-class mothers thought of child abuse when seeing video clips of Nso caretakers moving ("shaking") the baby up and down (Keller, 2022a).

Nso village babies are expected to listen carefully and not to contribute their own speech contributions. They are not entitled to address adults but only answer questions directed to them with short answers, mainly "yes" or "no". Nonverbal communication, on the other hand, is very sophisticated, based on observation and imitation as the major learning tools. This socialization strategy and learning environment adhere to the cultural model of hierarchical relatedness/action autonomy (Schröder et al., 2013).

Babies in urban middle-class families belonging to the non-WEIRD world learn a complex mixture of individually centered and communal orientations at the same time. Therefore, the cultural emphases are broadly distributed between self-enhancing strategies like face-to-face contact and individualized talk and community-fostering strategies based on the integration into a larger social network. The emphasis at the same time on a communal and individual understanding of the self allows children to develop an integrated understanding of self that is able to pursue self-interests but naturally also adopts responsibilities for others. This autonomous-related self (Kagitcibasi, 2017; Keller, 2012a) also allows switching between contexts

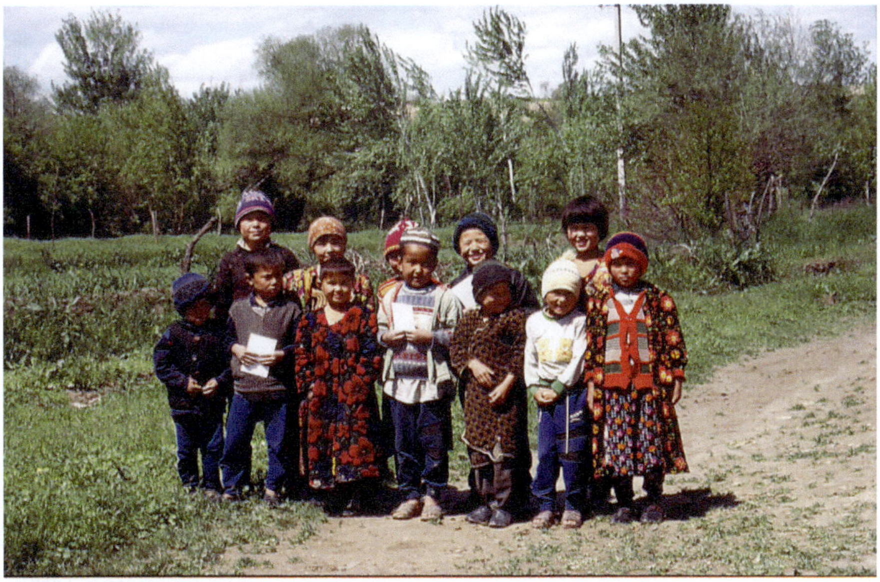

FIGURE 5 Children close to Samarkand. Copyright Kristin Moritz

with different contextual requirements. This socialization strategy and learning environment adhere to the combined cultural model of psychological autonomy/hierarchical relatedness.

The different socialization strategies are mirrored in children's development, with earlier or later achievements (e.g., Keller & Kärtner, 2013) and different phenotypical appearances.

Notes

1 See Ndzenyuiy and Keller (2025).
2 Thanks for the help from Prof. Nandita Chaudhary in composing this portrait.

6

IMPLICATIONS FOR CULTURE-CONSCIOUS RESEARCH

Abstract

Comparisons of developmental achievements across cultures are much more complicated than the usual practice of comparing the same behavior at the same time across different samples conveys. This standard procedure necessarily leads to wrong results and unjustified interpretations. It is argued that the specification of culture has consequences for design and samples. Designs need to take different cultural emphases for different achievements into account. This implies assessing the cultural emphases as well and contextualizing achievements instead of just treating them as variables. Samples cannot just be random collections of participants from countries, but need to be conceptually based. It is argued that homogeneous samples along sociodemographic characteristics are preferable for cross-cultural comparisons, since random samples or even representative samples (if they are possible at all) can mask cultural differences. It is demonstrated that the assessment of meaning systems is also important for studying samples belonging to the same cultural milieu, since there may be different components that cause variability.

Comparing a particular developmental achievement at the same time across different groups relating to different cultural models necessarily leads to advantages for one group and disadvantages for others. The disadvantages often apply to the traditional rural farming communities, since most of the research is biased toward WEIRD populations. Even if the superiority of non-WEIRD babies in a developmental achievement is recognized, the language use nevertheless refers to the WEIRD standard. Thus, the obvious

DOI: 10.4324/9781003672050-7

superiority of gross motor achievements of traditional farmer babies is not described as superiority in the literature, but as precocity (Keller, 2010), i.e., occurring at a time when it is untimely. Differences in favor of WEIRD babies are interpreted as deficiencies in non-WEIRD babies and serve as a rationale for many intervention activities, which will be discussed later. In order to be fair, designs therefore need to take different cultural emphases into account. This implies that meaning systems necessarily need to be assessed and considered for the interpretation of data.

This is also relevant for predictions of behavioral achievements, which might be better based on the meaning systems of caregivers than on the behaviors of children. In our research program, we found repeatedly that socialization goals of caregivers were better predictors of children's achievements than children's preceding behaviors (Keller & Kärtner, 2013). In order to get a more accurate picture, we tried to pair different developmental achievements that were differently emphasized in different cultural environments, like self-recognition (priority in WEIRD communities) and self-regulation (priority in traditional farming communities) (Keller et al., 2004) in order to balance the design and avoid misperceptions of deficit views. Cultural comparative research is obviously much more complicated than mainstream research suggests.

Using stimulus material that has been developed in one cultural community needs to be appropriated for cultural suitability when applied in other cultural communities in order to ensure comparability. The cultural appropriation needs to go beyond equivalence and bias control that quantitative cross-cultural methodology suggests (He & van de Fijver, 2012).

In a comparative study on memory development in Nso village children and German middle-class children, we wanted to use one of these tasks where objects have to be memorized as located in differently colored drawers of a box. Our Nso collaborators informed us that this task would not work with Nso children. Using a memory box with many finely differentiated colors could be problematic, as some drawers could not be reliably distinguished or consistently labeled. Our Cameroonian Co-PI, Dr. Relindis Yovsi, explained

> While Lamnso[1] has lexicalized terms for many colours, everyday discourse tends to reduce the colour spectrum into broader categories. Four dominant groups emerge:
>
> - White (fevir) – A distinct, culturally salient color.
> - Black (sen) – Encompasses not only black but also darker hues such as blue, green, and purple. This suggests a semantic extension where darkness, depth, or opacity are the core meaning.

- Red (baar) – Covers bright, warm shades including orange, (*woren-woren*), yellow (*she/sheshén*), and pink (*ping*). The unifying feature here is brightness or vividness, not the precise hue.
- Neutral/Residual (biibii, kibvekibve) – Brown and grey are acknowledged but often treated as "neutral" or less sharply categorized. This reflects a secondary status compared to primary contrasts of light/dark and bright/dull.

> In Lamnso, *fevir (white)*, *sen (black)*, and *baar (red)* function as basic prototypes, while other colour terms are either extensions or loan-influenced additions. The prominence of *sen* (black) to cover multiple dark colours may connect to environmental references (night, soil, deep water, shadows). Similarly, *baar* (red) grouping all bright shades could be tied to fire, blood, or ripe fruit as cultural anchors. Terms like *ping* and *poper* show lexical borrowing from English, reflecting modern contact and the need to name non-traditional colour categories. Forms like *worènworèn* (orange) and *kibvekibve* (grey) use reduplication, a common African linguistic strategy for intensification, descriptiveness, or approximation.
>
> *(Yovsi, personal communication, 2025)*

Differentiated color lexica have been reported from other cultures as well. Some languages have more or fewer basic color terms, like the Berinmo from Papua New Guinea. This language has five basic color terms, which don't directly map onto English categories. For example, they may group colors English speakers see as distinct (like green and blue) into one category. Another example are the Himba in Namibia, who use a different set of color categories, making it hard to distinguish between certain colors (e.g., blue and green), yet they are more sensitive to differences within what we might call "green". It is apparent that particularly the differentiation between green and blue is difficult in many cultures (for more information, see, e.g., Wierzbicka, 1990).

The same methodology, therefore, cannot be applied across cultural environments without producing artifacts that are, moreover, ethical transgressions when the results are interpreted as deficits. Nevertheless, it has been very difficult to convince journal reviewers that comparability of results needs to be based on cultural content, which may imply quite different phenotypical appearances.

Also, research strategies can be more or less culturally appropriate. WEIRD protocols assume as taken for granted that individuals can decide on their own whether they want to participate in a research project or not. It is further assumed that knowledge is an individual possession, where every owner is entitled to share it or not with whomever they want. Yet the decider and owner of knowledge may not be the individual who is subject to the study, but rather an authority from the family or household. In one of our cross-cultural studies, we wanted to assess ethnotheories of young mothers about socialization goals and childrearing beliefs in different cultural communities. This worked fine in European and Euro-American middle-class families, yet got us into trouble, e.g., in rural families in Gujarat, India. Whenever we approached a young mother, her husband or the mother-in-law intervened and answered the questions, since the young mothers were not entitled to share this knowledge with strangers. It was a major learning experience to understand that our research design was a transgression and an insult to the community's morals.

Thus, knowledge is a communal possession in rural traditional contexts, yet there is a distinct etiquette about the dissemination. This is different from the communal possession of objects, as we learned from a Nso grandmother. We asked her who owns the rubber shoes placed in front of the house. She was confused by the question and did not understand what these strangers wanted to know. She finally said, whoever needs the shoes uses them.

Using a research protocol that has been developed in WEIRD contexts may be ignorant of local realities. In our earlier cross-cultural research program, we assessed statements concerning socialization goals for early childhood in a Likert-like format, mainly from totally agree to totally disagree on a seven-point scale. This format worked well in middle-class families, irrespective of cultural background. More or less by chance, we found out that one of our Cameroonian research assistants, working in villages in the Northeastern grassfields, had changed the rating scale into a yes/no format. Overcoming the initial dismay about lacking equivalence of methods, we understood that our research assistant was responding sensitively to the local culture, which does not build on this kind of differentiated choices. By applying a rating scale format, she did not act in accordance with the cultural standards of the community. Choice generally is a WEIRD conception that is based on contextual and cultural prerequisites (see, e.g., Rosenfeld, 2025; Markus & Schwartz, 2010) that are not applicable globally. Thus, by not following the protocol, our research assistant helped us understand the cultural conception of decision-making in this community. We developed together a pairwise comparison format instead, where every item was compared to every other one with a yes or no decision (Keller & Kärtner, 2013).

Gabriel Scheidecker (2025) made similar observations in his field research in Madagascar. He got the impression in interviews that the mothers expressed quite similar perspectives. Even between the models of mothers and babysitters, contrary to his initial expectation, no fundamental differences emerged.

After only a few interviews in Ranomadio, this fact had already led his research assistants to the opinion that further interviews were not necessary, since one could already anticipate the answers.

In our research program about self-development across cultures, we studied mirror recognition across cultural communities (Kärtner et al., 2012). We found ourselves confronted with the question of a reviewer of a paper asking why we did not use the same size mirrors in German middle-class families and Indian Gujarati villagers. In German middle-class families, we used mirrors, in which children could see their whole bodies. Yet, our procedure had to take into account the different popularity of mirrors in the everyday life of families and children. In the rural Gujarati families, small mirrors, if at all, were only placed on higher boards close to the Hindu home worshiping altar and were mainly out of the sight of children.[2] Therefore, we used smaller mirrors, in which the children could see their faces. Yet there is pressure from journals and reviewers to apply the same methods, which obviously are inappropriate for a particular context.

The statistical treatment of biases to establish equivalence (see, e.g., He & Van de Fijver, 2012) often falls short when the assessment situation is already culturally biased, e.g., children are placed in a face-to-face situation with adults, possibly even in a separate room, which is not only not their everyday reality, but also a culturally inappropriate setting. Attachment researchers particularly insist on the scenario of standardized methodology when conducting the Strange Situation Procedure in non-WEIRD environments (see Mesman et al., 2016).

Thus, taking culture and cultural differences seriously has massive implications for research designs and the selection of samples. Obviously, assessing behavior at the same time in different samples with the same or superficially adapted methods across cultures is the wrong strategy.

Samples also cannot be just convenient or a random group of people living in one country, but need to be conceptually grounded. Randomly composed samples may include participants belonging to different environmental milieus and therefore represent different cultural models. Consequently, different randomly composed country samples are inappropriate to study cultural differences. Also, research that is not geared at cultural comparisons needs to specify for whom the sample stands. There is no such thing as a universal participant who is representative of the world's population as a whole, as we have already argued in Chapter 1.

Therefore, it is advocated here for homogeneous samples, i.e., participants should be similar to each other in critical variables or dimensions, especially the sociodemographic dimensions. Yet, it is important to stress again that the results based on homogeneous samples only relate to the population for which the sample stands.

The claim for representative samples in mainstream research serves the philosophy of universality. Maybe the popular discussion about the replication crisis in psychology, i.e., the difficulty in reproducing the results of many published psychology studies, leading to concerns about the reliability and validity of psychological research (Wiggins & Christopherson, 2019), may also have its roots in different sample compositions.

But even homogeneous samples contain variability. Samples that possess the same sociodemographic profile may be composed of participants with different family backgrounds, e.g., single parents, patchwork families, different sibling status (e.g., first born, second born, single child), different family traditions (e.g., celebrating holidays and family cohesion), being more or less socially integrated (having friends and community-based alliances), more or less successful (career orientation), and much more, which all may influence the behavior and the representations that they contribute to research studies. Religion, e.g., is mostly assessed in non-WEIRD samples as a sample characteristic; interestingly, much less is reported in WEIRD studies. Its intensity is only assessed if it is the topic of the study. Yet, religiosity, especially its intensity, may have an essential influence, particularly on issues of children's learning environments.

Moreover, cultural models that are associated with sociodemographic profiles cover diverse dimensions that may be differently popular in different samples with the same sociodemographic profile and cultural model. For example, Dutch and US American middle-class samples of parents that both represent WEIRD contexts differed in their ethnotheories of childrearing as outlined by Super and Harkness. Dutch parents emphasized more egalitarian and autonomy-supportive practices, fostering independence and self-regulation in children, whereas US Euro–American parents often focus on nurturing individual achievement and emotional expressiveness. All these dimensions support psychological autonomy in a broader sense, yet accentuate different dimensions through differing parenting strategies (Harkness et al., 2000). Whether this is challenging the "Western mind", as these authors propose, is open to debate. Also, Keller and Demuth (2005) found differences between two sociodemographically similar samples (Euro-American and German middle class), both adhering to psychological autonomy as a socialization goal. The participants did have a different understanding of the importance of different caregiving practices. German participants shared a holistic view in that they expected breastfeeding, body contact, and Beschäftigung ("dealing with the child") all to serve the development of psychological closeness and stimulation that are considered necessary for healthy development. Los Angeles mothers and grandmothers share a functionalistic view in that they expected different caregiving practices to have different developmental outcomes (breastfeeding is for health, playing is for stimulating cognitive development, bodily proximity is for soothing).

This necessary change of perspective in conducting cultural/cross-cultural research is also important for the applied field because it is inextricably interrelated with basic science. Applied programs are expected to be scientifically grounded and evidence-based. Therefore, it is important to decompose applied approaches and programs in order to uncover explicit and implicit assumptions. Attachment theory will be a case in point to exemplify these issues.

Notes

1 Lamnso is the local language of the Nso.
2 The familiarity with mirrors did not affect the mirror self-recognition.

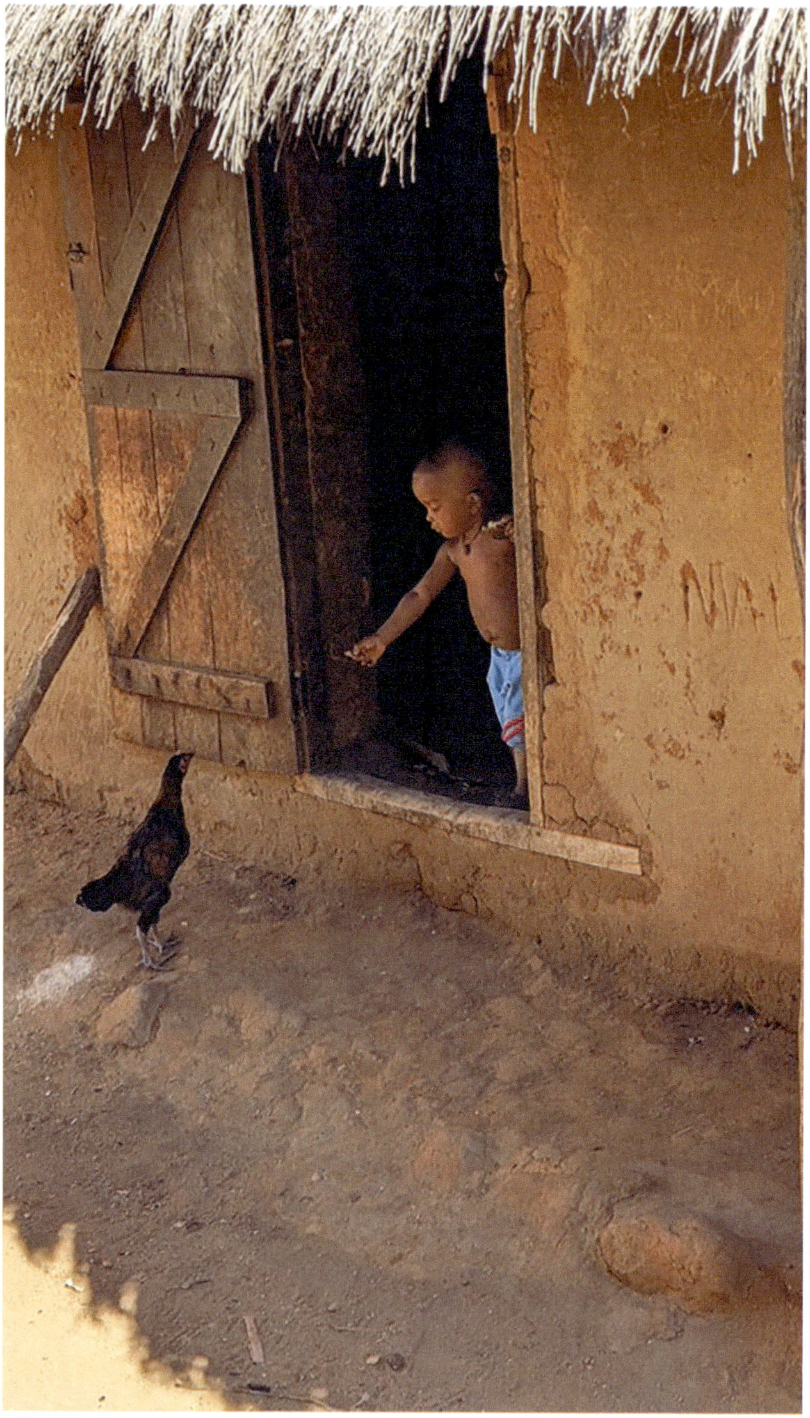

FIGURE 6 Child in Menamaty, southern Madagascar. Copyright Gabriel Scheidecker

PART 2

Attachment theory

Science and reality

7

HISTORY AND CORE ASSUMPTIONS OF ATTACHMENT THEORY

Abstract

In this paragraph, a brief account of the history and the core assumptions of attachment theory will be outlined. We refer to the origins of attachment theory, as formulated by John Bowlby and supplemented by Mary Ainsworth, as a conception of early socio-emotional development and its role as an organizer of following developmental pathways. This conception is still part of current curricula. Later additions of attachment theory, like intergenerational transmission, the life span approach, romantic relationships, and many others, are not considered, mainly because they are not relevant for the applied fields that are addressed in this book.

The problems of the definitions, assumptions, and the explicit and implicit implications will be outlined. It is obvious that the vagueness and fuzziness, and even the incorrectness, of many taken-for-granted assumptions challenge the scientific value of attachment theory substantially.

7.1 The origins and history of attachment theory

Attachment theory was founded by the British psychoanalyst and child psychiatrist Edward John Mostyn Bowlby (1907–1990). Bowlby practiced in the London Tavistock Hospital during the post-World War II era. Observing children who had experienced trauma and loss led him to question the psychoanalytic focus on intrapsychic conflicts and instead emphasize behavioral dynamics, particularly in the family. Also, his personal experiences may

DOI: 10.4324/9781003672050-9

have stimulated his interest in the consequences of trauma and loss. He was born into an upper-middle-class family where children were mainly raised by nannies. His nanny, to whom he had a close relationship, left the family when he was three years old, which obviously left traces in his psyche. His major focus on separation certainly was based on his clinical and personal experiences. Bringing together what he understood from different disciplines like primatology, ethology, evolutionary theories, and system theory, he composed a conception of children's early socio-emotional development centering around the child's relationship to a primary caregiver, which was more and more centered around the biological mother (Bowlby, 1986).

The second founding person of this conception was Mary Dinsmore Salter Ainsworth (1913–1999), a Canadian/US psychologist, who started working with John Bowlby in London during the 1950s. Influenced by her PhD supervisor William Blatz's security theory, which emphasized the importance of secure dependency for children to explore new challenges, Ainsworth's early work focused on familial security, though her main contributions to attachment theory can be viewed as secondary to Bowlby's foundational ideas (although many attachment researchers see her contribution as equally important as Bowlby's). While she expanded on topics like individual differences in attachment, sensitivity, and the attachment–exploration balance – key concepts already present in Bowlby's writings – her primary legacy is the invention of the Strange Situation Procedure (SSP), a laboratory-based observation protocol of mother, child, and a stranger in different combinations (see Ainsworth et al., 1978) to assess differences in attachment qualities. Her initial ethnographic methodology, combining interviews with naturalistic observations first in Uganda and later in Baltimore, US, was replaced by the SSP by following attachment researchers. Mary Ainsworth is reported to have expressed regret that the SSP overshadowed her earlier naturalistic fieldwork – particularly her Uganda (Ganda) project. It took away the attention of feeding, close bodily contact, face-to-face play, crying in the home, or just plain mother–infant patterns, so that she concluded

> … that so many attachment researchers have gone on to do research with the Strange Situation rather than looking at what happens in the home or in other natural settings.....it marks a turning away from „field work", and I don't think it's wise.
>
> *(Ainsworth & Marvin, 1995, p. 12)*

However, the success story seems to have allayed her concerns (Karen, 1994) (for more detailed accounts of the origins of attachment theory, see Duschinsky, 2020).

Over the about 60 years of history of attachment theory, different generations have left their footprints. The first (Bowlby, Ainsworth) and second generations (e.g., Main, Sroufe, Egeland) were very defensive of the original ideas and assumptions. Duschinsky reports that "looking back with regret, Waters jokingly characterized Sroufe, himself and other members of Ainsworth's circle as like a squad of Huns riding into battle whenever a threat was sensed". A third generation is obviously overcoming the defensive attitude of first- and second-generation researchers and adding a new twist to the discussion. Duschinsky (2025) conceives of generations not by chronological age. He uses the concept of generation pragmatically to characterize members of a cohort who, facilitated by structural factors that suggest commonalities, regard themselves as facing a bundle of common challenges, including delimitation and appraisal of the legacy of an earlier generation. He sees a third generation of attachment researchers constituted by the playing out of problems in theory and method.

> Madigan, Fearon, and colleagues recommended that attachment researchers should now seek to refocus on mechanisms, entering into dialogue with other disciplines, with methods such as the Strange Situation used as a tool rather than guiding the direction of research and sequestering researchers from this wider scientific conversation.
>
> *(Duschinsky, 2025)*

This openness is a major change in attitude. It remains to be seen the extent to which this lack of defensiveness and open door will be fully achieved.

Detailed and thoughtful discussions of the history of attachment theory and the different representatives over the generations can be found, e.g., in Duschinsky (2020, 2025), van der Horst (2011a,b), Bretherton (1992), and Vicedo (2013).

7.2 What is attachment?

Attachment theory is certainly one of the most popular conceptions in developmental psychology and related fields. It is one of the most iridescent conceptions at the same time, despite the popular understanding that attachment researchers talk and write about the same thing and understand each other (Schuengel et al., 2013; Fearon & Schuengel, 2021). This applies even more strongly to the applied field. A closer inspection, however, uncovers this view as an illusion.

Zentner (2025) talks about attachment Platonism in this respect. It expresses the preference for a clear and undisturbed idea over the contradictions of reality. The reality Zentner has in mind is that different assessment tools of attachment security do not produce largely overlapping results. For example, Cadman et al. (2017) demonstrated in a meta-analysis that the Strange Situation and the Attachment Q-sort (Waters & Deane, 1985), the two most prominent procedures to assess attachment security, only correlate r = .25, thus basically assessing different phenomena. He identifies Platonism as a general principle in psychology, which is especially prominent in the attachment discourse.

Therefore, based on the existing conceptual information and the empirical evidence, it is not easy to define attachment and describe attachment theory as a unitary conception. The problems are located on several levels. It already starts with John Bowlby's writings. Basic terms are ill defined, and conceptions from other domains are wrongly interpreted (see Keller, 2022a). He held different positions in different writings and used several definitions for the same term (Duschinsky, 2020). The vagueness and inexactness opened the floor for the interpretations of the following attachment researchers. Duschinsky (2025) demonstrated in a meticulous analysis that there are differences in the understanding of attachment and its constituent terms among different schools and generations of attachment researchers. There are moreover different discourses in different domains, like popular discourses, developmental science, social psychological science, psychiatric diagnosis, psychotherapy, and child welfare practice (Duschinsky et al., 2021). Also, the diversity in the use of attachment concepts across different domains of application has been largely unrecognized. Wrong interpretation, wrong usage, and simplification are widespread (e.g., Forslund et al., 2021). Nevertheless, there is a general understanding in science and application that attachment theory is a clean and coherent theory (e.g., Thompson, 2026).

The most common definition in science as well as practice is that attachment is an emotional bond. However, the understanding of what an emotional bond is can vary widely. Kindergarten teachers, who were asked to draw attachment as an emotional bond, came up with very different interpretations, from abstract patterns to depictions of hearts, hands, and people (see Keller, 2022a, p. 26). In the applied field, there is often also confusion about whether attachment refers to the emotional connection or affection a child develops toward a caregiver (what Bowlby's original intention was) or to the caregiver's emotional bond to the child. The focus on the early maternal–infant bond had been strongly influenced by two pediatricians, Marshall Klaus and John Kennell, in the 1970s. They proposed that the hours immediately after birth are critical, during which close contact between mother and newborn fosters emotional bonding of the mother to her baby, which has lasting impacts on maternal behavior and consequently on child development. They observed that mothers who had early, uninterrupted skin-to-skin contact with their babies soon after birth seemed to be more responsive and nurturing. These mothers were more likely to breastfeed longer, show affectionate behaviors, and report stronger feelings of attachment (Klaus & Kennell, 1976).

Although replications revealed mixed results and their conception was criticized, Klaus and Kennell helped humanize childbirth by emphasizing the emotional needs of both mother and baby. Their advocacy shifted practices from cold, clinical routines toward more compassionate, relationship-centered care (e.g., rooming in).

Another interpretation of emotional bond, which was also visualized in the kindergarten teachers' drawings, represented ribbons, ropes with two ends, capturing the mutual relationship between two people. As these teachers all belonged to the German middle class, they thought of attachment naturally as a dyadic bond.

Besides the emotional bond, Bowlby offers a second definition of attachment in his writings: attachment as a behavioral system, based on ethology, namely an innate behavioral system in infants that ensures proximity to caregivers (usually the mother) for survival and protection. The attachment system is activated in situations of stress or threat, prompting the infant to seek closeness to the caregiver, including behaviors like crying, clinging, and following, which serve to maintain contact with the caregiver (Duschinsky, 2020).

The two concepts – attachment behavior and emotional attachment – are not the same, but they have often been blurred in interpretations of Bowlby's theory. Duschinsky (2020) argues that this conceptual ambiguity has led to confusion in research, clinical practice, and public discourse.

Following generations of attachment researchers have added to and expanded attachment theory, e.g., by extending it to a life span approach, including attachment representations of adults, romantic relationships, intergenerational transmission, neurocognition, and more. Ross Thompson (2017) talks about the attachment theory of the 21st century as a roof under which many mini attachment theories have been assembled. Nevertheless, the confusion remains part of attachment research. The roof does not represent an overarching perspective. Duschinsky (2025) argues that the mini-theories did not clarify their exact premises, their respective agreements or disagreements with Bowlby, their perceptions of the strengths or weaknesses of his ideas, their respective agreements or disagreements with one another, and their specific implications for practice.

In conclusion, Duschinsky ends the epilogue of his 2025 book with:

> In contrast to the impression from cut-price versions in ready circulation, attachment research is not a single whole; there are important vectors of current development and debate. Perception of this diversity is essential for understanding its interest and its value.

The discussion in this book is restricted to the original conception, i.e., relationship formation during the first years (Bowlby, 1969). Although attachment researchers continue claiming tremendous changes over time (e.g., Thompson, 2017; Foster et al., 2025), the assumptions about early attachment formation have not changed much, as will be demonstrated in the following. Where some movement can be recognized is in the identity of the attachment figure. In the beginning, Bowlby talked about the family, which boiled down to the mother thereafter and the assumption of monotropy (for a discussion, see Keller, 2022a). Monotropy is understood as the **one special, primary attachment** to a main caregiver, mainly the biological mother, which is considered more significant than any other person. The assumption of monotropy has been discarded theoretically, so that other attachment figures can be considered primary attachment figures. In reality, however, it is mainly the mother who is participating in attachment assessments and in practical applications, like parenting interventions.

Central to the early attachment formation are emerging differences in attachment quality. Ainsworth formalized three different attachment strategies based on her observational studies, including the 1953–1955 Uganda research and the subsequent Baltimore project (1967; Ainsworth et al., 1978). She differentiated secure, insecure avoidant, and insecure ambivalent attachment strategies, which were later complemented by Mary Main (Main & Solomon, 1986) with the conception of disorganized attachment. Secure and the two types of insecure attachment strategies are considered related to the caregiver's sensitivity, defined as the prompt, consistent, adequate reaction to the infant's signals. Disorganized attachment is regarded more as a pathological condition that emerges from childhood experiences of trauma or neglect (for more details, see below).

It is this conception that also has a special impact in some applied fields, like family court decisions (see also Zentner, 2025). In the following, the basic assumptions of attachment theory will be summarized, followed by a critical evaluation and discussion of these assumptions.

7.3 The basic assumptions of attachment theory

7.3.1 Attachment is an innate biological system

It is assumed that humans are born with a biological drive to form attachments to one or a few caregivers, which evolved in the savannah environment of the early human hunter-gatherers, the "Environment of Evolutionary Adaptedness" (EEA), a term coined by psychologist John Tooby and anthropologist Leda Cosmides (1992) in the context of evolutionary theories. They emphasized the importance of understanding this context to comprehend modern human behavior and cognition.

This environment contained many challenges for babies such as predators, temperature changes, and an insecure physical environment, which could be reduced by a protective adult. Attachment thus serves a survival function by keeping the child close to a protective adult.

7.3.2 The attachment system becomes activated under distress

The attachment system starts working automatically when the child feels insecure, is distressed, and/or uneasy. It is expressed through attachment behaviors like crying, clinging, following, and reaching out, which should secure the caregiver's attention and care and serve comforting functions.

It is assumed that children are also born with an exploration drive that regulates learning and information processing. Attachment and exploration are seen as antagonistic systems: the exploration system is active when the attachment system is inactive, and vice versa. This relationship is fundamental to the application of attachment theory in early education and pedagogics. Children who are occupied with attachment work are oriented exclusively to the attachment figure who serves as a secure base or secure haven. The concept of a "secure base" refers to a reliable and trustworthy figure, typically a caregiver, mainly the mother, who provides a sense of safety and security to a child. This secure base allows the child to explore the environment and develop independence, knowing that he/she can return to the caregiver for support, comfort, and reassurance. The implications for the caregiver are:

Availability: The caregiver is consistently present and responsive to the child's needs, providing emotional support during times of stress or fear, thus reducing the attachment needs.

Trust and Stability: The caregiver's consistent behavior creates a sense of stability and trust, enabling the child to feel secure in his/her relationship so that exploration is triggered.

7.3.3 Caregiver sensitivity influences attachment security

Caregiver sensitivity plays a crucial role in the formation of attachment security in children. It refers to the ability of a caregiver to perceive, interpret, and respond immediately, appropriately, and consistently to a child's signals and needs. This includes being attuned to the child's emotional state, understanding the cues (such as crying, cooing, or gestures), and responding in a nurturing and consistent manner even to the most subtle infant signal. Consistency is important for children's belief that they can rely on their caregivers. The sensitive responsiveness should prime children to feel understood and valued, fostering a sense of safety and security. This is the assumed basis for the development of secure attachment. Inconsistent, neglectful, or intrusive caregiving, on the other hand, can result in insecure attachment styles (e.g., anxious, avoidant, disorganized). Caregiver's sensitivity can be affected by the caregiver's own stress levels and emotional availability. A caregiver dealing with high stress or emotional difficulties may struggle with responsiveness, which can lead to insecure attachments.

Mary Ainsworth defined sensitivity on a 9-point scale, leading from complete sensitivity to complete insensitivity.[1] To receive the highest score on the sensitivity scale necessitates exclusive 24/7 attention, which Bowlby in some of his writings demanded (Duschinsky, 2020).

Caregiver sensitivity is considered a foundational aspect of attachment security in children. Parents and caregivers who foster these qualities are assumed to create the conditions for children to develop strong, healthy relationships throughout their lives.

7.3.4 Early attachment experiences shape internal working models

Attachment quality at about one year develops into an internal representation over the next two to three years, the Internal Working Model. Bowlby understood it as a system of thoughts, convictions, expectations, emotions, and behaviors concerning the self and others resulting from previous social experiences.

The model is often considered a cognitive framework or a mental representation that influences how individuals see themselves, understand relationships, interpret social interactions, and navigate emotional experiences throughout their lives. The IWM is the basis for relationships between attachment qualities and the later developmental course.

These basic assumptions are based on more general principles. The most encompassing principle is the principle of universality. Universality is a foundational concept of attachment theory, simply stating that all aspects of attachment theory are universal. It posits that all human beings, regardless of culture or background, have an innate capacity to form attachment relationships with caregivers if there is no neurophysiological damage, and that attachment has the same meaning, emerges in the same way, and has the same consequences across cultures and contexts. Universality is bound to the principle of normativity, indicating that in contexts that are not life-threatening, most children will develop *secure attachment* relationships. With this, it is also assumed to be the best for children's healthy and happy development and is taken as the typical or default pattern. Many attachment theorists argue that secure attachment would represent the adaptation that emerged during the EEA. This assumption is based on empirically assessed distributions of attachment qualities, mainly with the SSP.

Ainsworth's Baltimore study distribution of about 66% secure (Type B), 12% avoidant (Type A), and 22% ambivalent/resistant (Type C) attachment strategies is regarded as the standard distribution. Global meta-analyses show similar overall proportions, though country-level deviations occur in some studies – for example, more avoidant classifications in Israel and more resistant classifications in Japan. In line with the universality assumption, deviations are usually explained post hoc by methodological problems or even by context and culture (see, e.g., the differences between the northern German (Bielefeld) and the southern German (Regensburg) samples in the Grossmann research program (Grossmann et al., 1981; see also Mesman et al., 2016).

STRANGE SITUATION PROCEDURE

The SSP is a laboratory-based observational protocol developed by Mary Ainsworth in the context of the Baltimore study to assess the quality of attachment between infants and their primary caregivers. This procedure is notable for its structured approach to evaluating how children respond to separations and reunions with their caregivers (for more background, see Keller, 2022a).

The Strange Situation consists of eight episodes of about three minutes each, typically lasting about 20 minutes overall, designed to elicit certain behaviors in the child. The episodes include:

1 **Initial Introduction:** The caregiver and child enter an unfamiliar playroom where a variety of toys are available.
2 **Free Play:** The child is encouraged to explore the playroom while the caregiver remains present. This is meant to observe how securely the child feels with their caregiver.
3 **Stranger's Introduction:** A stranger enters the room, first talking to the caregiver and then interacting with the child. This helps assess the child's reaction to the stranger while the caregiver is present.
4 **Caregiver Leaves:** The caregiver quietly leaves the room, which assesses the child's reaction to separation (e.g., crying, distress, or indifference).
5 **Stranger Comforts:** The stranger stays with the child, observing how the child behaves when comforted by someone unfamiliar.
6 **Caregiver Returns:** The caregiver returns to the room and greets the child. This reunion is critical for assessing attachment behavior, including whether the child seeks comfort from the caregiver.
7 **Caregiver Leaves Again:** The caregiver leaves the child alone in the room once more, and the child's response to this separation is observed again.
8 **Caregiver Returns Again:** The caregiver returns to the room, and researchers observe the child's reaction to this final reunion.

Mainly based on children's behavior in the reunion episodes with the mother, Ainsworth identified three primary attachment styles:

9 **Secure Attachment:** Children with secure attachment typically show distress when separated from their caregiver but are easily comforted when they return. They feel safe exploring the environment.
10 **Insecure Avoidant Attachment:** These children tend to avoid or ignore the caregiver, and they often show little emotion when the caregiver leaves or returns. They might not seek comfort from the caregiver.

11 **Insecure Ambivalent (or Resistant) Attachment:** Children display intense distress when separated and exhibit clingy behavior. However, upon the caregiver's return, they may both seek and resist comfort, demonstrating confusion over how to react.

Later, Mary Main introduced a fourth category:

12 **Disorganized Attachment:** Characterized by a lack of a clear attachment behavior, these children may exhibit contradictory behaviors and appear dazed or confused. This style has often been associated with trauma or inconsistent caregiving. This happens when a child's need for safety conflicts with a caregiver's frightening or unpredictable behavior, leaving the child without a clear strategy for how to cope with their distress and leading to a pattern of confusing, contradictory behaviors.

The attachment quality is regarded as predicting later behavioral outcomes.

7.4 Critical evaluation of the core assumptions

The core assumptions leave many questions open concerning their scientific credibility and validity. The universality assumption is justified with the assumed evolutionary origin of attachment. However, how evolutionary theory is interpreted in Bowlby's and many other attachment researchers' writings is highly problematic. Although there are many versions and interpretations of evolutionary theories (e.g., Levit et al., 2008), there are some core assumptions that are relevant. One important one is that evolution does not have a goal or intentional direction, except for optimal reproductive success. It is a natural process that occurs through mechanisms such as mutation, natural selection, genetic drift, and gene flow. These mechanisms lead to changes in populations over time, but they do not imply a specific psychological or social aim or purpose. Evolution is a response to environmental pressures and changes, operating with the principle of variation within populations rather than having a preset goal or end state.

Another important point is that the environment plays a critical role in shaping the evolutionary process by exerting selective pressures on the population level. Adaptations to the particular environment, the ecosocial context, enhance survival and reproductive success in specific environments. Some anthropologists and psychologists (Belsky et al., 1991; Chisholm, 1999) had identified different developmental pathways to reproductive success along these lines. They differentiated a quantitative and a qualitative reproductive strategy. The more quantitative strategy described a developmental pathway with children being raised in an unpredictable, insecure, low-resource family environment, where children possibly develop insecure relationships, start sexual relations early, change partners often, become parents early, and demonstrate low parental investment themselves. The qualitative strategy refers to children coming from a stable family of origin, having developed secure attachment relationships, starting relatively late but having more enduring sexual relationships, starting comparatively later with their own reproduction, and becoming highly investing parents. Both strategies are equal from an evolutionary perspective since different environments promote different strategies to reach optimal reproductive success. Therefore, from an evolutionary perspective, one conception cannot be superior to another conception in psychological terms. Evolutionary theories do not deal with well-being, trust, or happiness. The currency is reproductive success, i.e., the optimal transmission of genes. Whether an individual is happy or unhappy, gets along well or not in life, is securely attached or not, does not play a role in this framework.

Yet, attachment theory clearly evaluates one strategy as supporting the development of secure attachment and thus a better life prospect, and one strategy as inferior, leading to insecure attachment and thus anticipating problematic life strategies.

Already the British ethologist Robert Hinde (1982), who was one of Bowlby's informants about ethological approaches, had critically remarked that natural selection does not favor a particular maternal strategy to foster secure attachment, like responsive sensitivity. The empirical relationship between sensitivity and attachment security is modest, as meta-analyses have revealed (e.g., already de Wolff & van IJzendoorn, 1997). De Wolff and van IJzendoorn (1997) analyzed 66 studies involving over 4,000 infants and found a positive correlation of r .24, which represents a small to moderate effect. They concluded that sensitivity matters, but other dimensions also play a role, like temperament or other characteristics of the caregiver's behavior. A more recent meta-analysis by Verhage et al. (2016) also found modest associations between sensitivity and attachment security. They also included intervention studies aimed at improving caregiver sensitivity, which showed stronger relations (see also van den Boom, 1997).

However, the strong relationships that Mary Ainsworth reported from her Baltimore study were never replicated again. Ainsworth found that sensitivity could predict attachment security with considerable accuracy (about 70% of the time). Yet, the quality of the home observations and their documentation raises substantial doubts about the quality of the assessment, as Marga Vicedo (2013) has concluded from her work with the raw data, including detailed observational notes, interview transcripts, and behavioral measures in the Murray Research Archive, affiliated with Harvard University's Murray Center Archive of the Baltimore study (for more details, see Keller, 2022a).

There are more arguments specifying a wrong understanding of evolutionary theories in attachment theory. Marga Vicedo discusses and articulates sophisticatedly the lacking building blocks needed to formulate an evolutionary account (2013, 2017a, b, 2018). She argues that the claim that attachment was an adaptation would imply that it was the result of natural selection. However, the principle of natural selection is to select between alternatives; it can only produce changes if there is a genetic base. Accordingly, there should be genes for children's proximity seeking and maternal sensitivity. Natural selection would favor carriers of these genes if they lead to better reproductive success. There are no studies proving this possibility. Looking more closely at this situation, it turns out to be even more complex. A behavior that has been adaptive during the past must not necessarily continue to be adaptive in a massively changed environment – or do we still have the Stone Age psychology, as the founder of human ethology, Irenäus Eibl-Eibesfeldt, thought even during the 1980s (Eibl-Eibesfeld, 2004)? Genetic changes can occur during short periods of time, e.g., the body size and the size of the beak of Galapagos finches changed during a short time span.

Marga Vicedo also argues against the concept of the EEA as the cradle of attachment for different reasons. The EEA is an unobservable, speculative construct based on inference rather than direct evidence, making it an unreliable foundation for understanding the origins of attachment. Attachment behaviors vary across cultures and historical periods, which challenges the idea that attachment systems evolved in response to a singular, uniform EEA. The EEA concept risks oversimplifying human evolution by reducing attachment to a rigid and static system, ignoring the complexity, plasticity, and dynamics of human attachment.

The conception of normativity is bound to the definition of a valid and reliable definition of attachment security, which does not reflect the empirical evidence. As Zentner's (2025) analysis has demonstrated, different tools obviously assess different things, since they do not overlap much. The evaluation of attachment security is therefore dependent on the instrument being used. Nevertheless, the Platonism effect overshadows the differences. This essentialism, as expressed in consistency and stability, is based on the conception of the Western mind as a bounded and predictable entity. However, in Buddhism, e.g., change is the essential principle of life. Zentner (2025) refers to the principle of impermanence (Liu et al., 2023), expressing that there is no essence or identity beyond the here and now. This implies that there is no stable core self across situations and times. Similar ideas are represented in personality psychology's trait-state distinction. Traits refer to consistent, stable characteristics or patterns of behavior, thoughts, and feelings that are relatively enduring over time and across different situations. Traits are thought to represent fundamental aspects of personality and are generally considered to be inherited or shaped early in life but can evolve slowly over time. States, on the other hand, refer to temporary, situational experiences or conditions that are typically influenced by immediate external circumstances. States can fluctuate widely based on the environmental affordances and constraints. Although there are individual and intracultural differences in trait and state orientation, there are tendencies of different intercultural preferences (Slabu et al., 2014).

The consequence of the assumptions of universality and normativity is the principle of competence. It relates the early attachment qualities to later developmental outcomes, first bound to the socio-emotional development, but soon extending to all developmental domains (see, e.g., Mikulincer & Shaver, 2021; for a critical discussion see Roisman & Groh, 2021). Securely attached children are assumed to fare better socio-emotionally and cognitively compared to insecurely attached children. The empirical examination of these assumed relationships is largely not convincing. British psychologist Elizabeth Meins discusses critically and profoundly the overestimation of the competence assumption in an opinion piece in *The Psychologist*, the organ of the British Society for Psychology (Meins, 2017). She expresses skepticism about attachment theory's prognostic value for all kinds of developmental results that are reported, reaching from brain development to behavioral disorders, including domains that cannot be related to attachment conceptually, like risky driving behavior or math achievements.

Zentner (2025) discusses three break points (Bruchstellen), as he calls them, of the competence hypothesis. The first is the positive effect of extrafamilial care. Attachment theory considers attachment as a specific relationship between an infant and a significant caregiver emerging during the first years of life and setting the stage for later development. The original assumption of monotropy, that there is only one significant caregiver, was later softened to a few significant caregivers. Yet the monotropy comes back in through the backdoor with the assumption of a hierarchy. There may be other people important for an infant, e.g., in terms of being favorite play partners (e.g., fathers), yet in terms of the primary attachment function, security and protection, it is the primary caregiver who is responsible.

Although theoretically any caregiving person can become the primary caregiver, in practice the mother is usually regarded as the primary attachment person. This is reflected in attachment research as well as in the applied field. There is some research with fathers and with day-care teachers – very few studies also assessed siblings as attachment figures. There are no studies assessing the attachment strategies to different caregivers as interrelated networks (see Keller, 2022a). If only the relationship with the significant caregiver could transmit the sense of security to the child to develop secure attachment, day care (out-of-home care) should have a disturbing effect, facilitating insecure attachment relationships. In fact, Bowlby warned that prolonged separation during the early years (especially before age three) could lead to emotional and social difficulties later in life (Bowlby, 1951). However, general negative effects could not be observed in the encompassing NICHD study (NICHD, 2001). There are, however, several studies demonstrating positive effects for socio-emotional and cognitive development (e.g., Melhuish et al., 2015).

Zentner's (2025) second break point concerns the lacking prognostic value of insecure attachment patterns. A large meta-theoretical analysis revealed no results regarding the predictive power of the two insecure classifications for externalizing problems. Children with a disorganized classification showed a minor relationship with externalizing behaviors (Fearon et al., 2010).

The third break point (Zentner, 2025) refers to possible alternative explanations. The mainly correlational attachment studies cannot reveal causal relationships. Genetic factors and multiple contextual influences can also prime particular behavioral expressions. The ignorance regarding alternative explanations has to do with the closed nature of confirmatory attachment research, especially in the first and second generations. The third generation seems to be more open in this respect, as discussed by Duschinsky (2025); see also Thompson, Simpson, and Berlin (2022).

Moreover, the long-term stability of attachment classifications is poor to non-existent (see, for a discussion, Zentner, 2025). In conclusion, attachment theory has serious conceptual problems with question marks on all the assumptions, principles, and taken-for-granted premises. An overarching problem is the ethnocentric nature of the assumptions. The most obvious ones will be introduced in the next chapter.

Note

1 http://www.psychology.sunysb.edu/attachment/measures/content/ainsworth_scales.html, Retrieved 2.3.2026.

8

THE ETHNOCENTRIC BIAS OF ATTACHMENT THEORY

Abstract

Attachment theory's assumptions and principles are based on taken-for-granted realities of a Western-centric, WEIRD worldview that sets the stage for children's learning environments. Accordingly, the WEIRD childcare philosophy reflects the conception of the person as a unique, separate, self-contained, i.e., psychologically autonomous person. The conception of the parent-child interaction as exclusively dyadic between an adult and a child, with the child's assumed wishes and intentions primacy, reflects the family milieu of the Western middle class. However, this childcare philosophy is not seen as a minority phenomenon, bound to specific contextual conditions, but is set as universal and normative, rendering other conceptions and models as deficient and in need of intervention and repair. Thus, the scientific questionability is complemented by ethical transgressions.

The WEIRD child's learning environment is built on a multitude of taken-for-granted pre-assumptions that are explicitly and implicitly built into the core assumptions and principles of attachment theory and the underlying philosophy of the Western middle-class ideal of humans. *It is taken for granted* that a child's caretaker must be an adult. Only adults are considered to be able to care for and supervise children for mainly two reasons. Children are not believed to be able to adequately assess risks and stimulate an infant. The second reason resonates with the conception of childhood as a protected time span, where children should not be assigned responsibility for the care and well-being of babies because they should not be restricted in their own activities like playing

DOI: 10.4324/9781003672050-10

and learning. There are legal regulations in many Western countries that prevent children from being alone with babies. Many migrant mothers living in Germany were confronted with youth services after they left a baby in the care of siblings in an apartment. Neighbors witnessing the situation call the youth service to prevent child abuse that they see in the situation. The protected childhood, on the other hand, alienates the child from the real everyday life and places him or her in a parallel world with strongly restricted learning opportunities. A closer observation of Western middle-class small children reveals that they, as babies from many communities worldwide (see below), are very much interested in other children, including other babies. Babies start crying when they hear other babies cry as an early contagious expression of empathy (Geangu et al., 2010). Thus, from birth on, children are interested in other children. They observe with keen interest what other children are doing. As much as they are told to be unique, they nevertheless also want to be like other children and fit in instead of sticking out.

Thus, the assumed inability to assess risks is a consequence of the segregated definition of childhood. If children are allowed to participate in the daily routines of a household or family, they learn to assess risks in situ. This is different in cultural environments where children participate in the ongoing everyday life, in which every member of the household, adult or child, participates. Lancy, e.g., has documented in an interesting paper that small children in many cultural environments of the majority world obviously handle machetes and big knives without notable accidents and without adult interference (Lancy, 2016; see also Keller, 2022a).

It is taken for granted that the attitude governing childcare is expected to be child-centered. However, what does child-centeredness mean? It is obviously defined by adults based on their interpretations of the child's assumed wishes/desires/intentions. These interpretations are more or less derived from attachment theoretic assumptions and their many versions. Although child-centeredness is supposed to be a sign of respect for children's autonomy, it actually undermines children's agency and its expressions (Alter & Raphael, 2024) since children are completely controlled by adults who navigate their world in an "illusion of autonomy" (Keller, 2012b). For example, adult caregivers formulate questions for their babies, offering them choices, like "do you want to play alone?", "do you want to sleep?", "do you want to see grandma tomorrow" and answer these questions based on their perception of mainly mimical infant signals, which is a merely subjective process. Certainly, an observer agreement about the meaning of infants' behavior related to a particular question could hardly be reached. In general, infants and toddlers largely depend on adults' definition of their environment and on their mediation of initiatives for peer contact, such as being taken to particular playgrounds, playdates, or day-care and educational institutions (Howes, 2009). In these spaces, adults not only design the environment but also structure activities, supervise, and directly intervene in peer interactions (Scheidecker, 2025).

Moreover, child-centeredness may have the opposite of its intended effect. Child-centeredness is supposed to prime children's autonomy. In fact, it also fosters children's dependence, because children become dependent on attention, especially exclusive attention devoted to them. They want to be watched whatever they do and expect unanimous praise for whatever they do. Thus, children hardly learn to negotiate spaces and limits between people but develop unrealistic self-perceptions and expectations (see, for example, Keller, 2022a).

It is taken for granted that babies and children need a special environment that is tailored to their assumed needs, in other words, that is child-friendly. On the one hand, children are considered competent information assessors and processors since the radical change of perspective from the brainless reflexive being (hirnrindenloses Reflexwesen, Scheler, 1927/2018) to the competent infant during the 1970s (Stone et al., 1973). On the other hand, they are assumed to be limited in their capacities to deal with stimulation, so that they should not be exposed to the usual family reality, but separated from the adult reality of daily life. The child-friendly environment is mainly indoors. Children have from birth their own room in which they should sleep alone as soon as possible. In general, they spend a lot of time alone because it is considered a need. If they spend social time, it is mainly one caregiver who is present. Mothers and fathers are taking turns (Keller, 2022a). The average time spent alone equals the time with a caregiver. On the other hand, toys are considered to be important for children, especially to stimulate their cognitive development. Toys should always be available within reach of children to provide a stimulating environment. Cognitive development is equated with brain development, with far-reaching consequences, extending into the state's economy and politics, as expressed in the ideology of intervention programs, discussed later.

So-called security blankets are soft toys/blankets that have a special emotional meaning for children and should function as replacements for an attachment figure. Many Western middle-class children need a particular (soft) object to calm down or fall asleep. Often, pacifiers are also crucial in this respect. Although many parents often do not approve of these objects, children's high-volume protest enforces their will. The weaning from a pacifier may become a painful process. In some German cities, there are pacifier trees, where parents bring their children to fix the pacifier in the tree while performing a mourning ritual like a funeral.

The question remains whether small children really want to spend time alone in the first place or want to manipulate their caregivers with their protest, as caregivers sometimes think. In any case, many questions about the interpretation of children's needs remain open.

Another taken-for-granted assumption is that children can be best stimulated and learn best in exclusive dyadic exchanges. Moreover, the adult partner is not random, so that children ought not to learn from any adult, but primarily from their caretakers or at least familiar persons. This philosophy can be seen particularly well in language learning/assessment research. In their influential word-gap study, Hart and Risley (1995, 2003) presented results that implied that there was a tremendous difference in the amount of child-directed speech between children from (socio)economically rather disadvantaged families and middle-class children of up to 30 million words over the first four years. The 1980 assessment of 42 families from Kansas, USA, consisted of a count of the words spoken to the child by the primary caregiver, who was, except in one case, the mother. The words were assessed with a recorder during one-hour weekly visits between the first and third birthdays. Out of these numbers, the number of words that the primary caregiver directed at the child was estimated for the first four years. The conclusion was finally based on comparing six children from disadvantaged families with 13 children from professional families. The results were never replicated and contain numerous methodological shortcomings. The restricted definition of children's language environment, excluding language directed to the child from other persons except the mother and ignoring the ambient language that a child is naturally exposed to, reflects the strength of presumptions (but see Miller et al., 2024; Ochs & Kremer-Sadlik, 2020).

The incredible success of this single, methodologically weak study in the applied field and its legitimation as the "scientific" base for numerous intervention programs from UNICEF to the Clinton Foundation confirms the appeal of simplicity. The estimation of socioeconomic group membership, based on formalized criteria (e.g., poverty estimations, see below), is sufficient to justify interventions without assessing the real situation, the circumstances, and especially the needs (Oppong & Strader, 2022).

It is a taken-for-granted assumption that the expression of emotions, and particularly positive emotions, is the default condition. Jeanne Tsai and colleagues (2007) argue that Euro-American research participants prefer high-arousal positive affective states, such as enthusiasm and excitement. Accordingly, the stimulation strategy of caregivers with infants, like high-pitched vocalizing and talking, and mimical exaggeration, is directed at increasing arousal to a peak (Keller, 2019). The expression of babies' positive emotions is reinforced and supported to continue. Positive emotions accentuate uniqueness and thus instantiate individuality (Shweder & Bourne, 1984).

Accompanying language reveals that the expression of positive emotions during interactional situations is interpreted as communication. Babies not smiling as their caregivers/mothers expect are suspected of expressing dissatisfaction with the interaction. One middle-class mother from Berlin commented on her failed attempts to get her three-month-old baby to smile in a research situation: "You already do not like mommy" (Keller, 2022a).

Negative emotions are stopped as soon as possible. However, caregivers first try to find out the reasons for crying by talking to the baby – "why are you crying?" – followed by checking hypotheses: "you can't be hungry", "are you tired?", "do you feel bored?" Changing the body position, increasing bodily closeness, and breastfeeding may follow, often with a considerable delay.

All these assumptions are derived from a childcare philosophy that reflects the WEIRD conception of the person as a unique, separated, self-contained, i.e., psychologically autonomous person who is supposed to pursue their self-interests with first priority. This childcare philosophy is set as universal. It is the soil in which attachment theory is planted. Ethnographic studies from other cultural communities, residing in other contextual conditions with other conceptions of the self, reveal the factual specificity of this socialization model, as apparent in the portraits (see above).

9

DIFFERENT AVENUES TO DEVELOP ATTACHMENT RELATIONSHIPS

Abstract

Attachment, i.e., close relationships during the first year, can obviously evolve through different channels. The Bowlby/Ainsworth view is that the perception of insecurity/anxiety elicits a biologically based system to ensure survival and development. They definitely deny the role of feeding/food as a relic of psychoanalytical dynamics. On the other hand, there is abundant evidence from ethnographic and cultural anthropological research that feeding and food are more than the intake of nourishment. Examples of different cultural contexts will be presented that demonstrate that food and feeding are building blocks of relations and bonding, deeply rooted in cultural meaning systems. A third avenue is identified in cultural learning. Cultural learning primes how children form close relationships by providing the models, routines, and meanings through which infants and caregivers interpret and respond to each other. This analysis demonstrates that not one entry pathway is normative, but that due to contextual variations, different entry pathways may be prevalent. It is also highly possible that the pathways are not exclusive, but interact and complement each other.

The Bowlby/Ainsworth view explains the drive for developing attachment as a biologically based system evolved to ensure survival and healthy (emotional) development in human infants. The attachment system is elicited through internal and external perceptions of insecurity, threat, and/or anxiety. John Bowlby rejected secondary drive theories, including psychoanalytic theories, which considered the child's motivation for attachment as derived from the gratification of hunger or libidinal drives related to the mother's

DOI: 10.4324/9781003672050-11

breast (Bowlby, 1958, 1980). Instead, he insisted that the mother–child bond is an independent psychological need that is not a result of associations with feeding (Bowlby, 1958; Cassidy, 2016; Van der Horst, 2011a, b). Bowlby saw empirical support for his assumptions in Harry F. Harlow and Robert R. Zimmermann's (1959) findings on surrogate rhesus macaque mothers (Blum, 2002) and concluded that "a newborn monkey will cling to a dummy provided it is soft and comfortable". The provision of food and warmth is quite unnecessary. Furthermore, "food plays only a marginal part in the development and maintenance of attachment behavior" (Bowlby, 1969, 224; see also Schmidt et al., 2023b; Funk et al., 2023; Scheidecker, 2025). He argued that instead of looking for food and gratification of physical needs, the infant seeks protection and safety in the caregiver's proximity (Bowlby, 1958, 1969; Cassidy, 2016). Mainstream attachment research in the following decades followed this view and barely investigated the critical attachment dynamics related to feeding. If feeding is addressed, most studies concentrate only on breastfeeding as an isolated variable and conclude that it is neither necessary nor sufficient to create infant–mother attachment, thereby concluding that feeding as a whole is not relevant for attachment (Colen & Ramey, 2014; Else-Quest et al., 2003; Peñacoba & Catala, 2019; Wilkinson & Scherl, 2006; see a review by Jansen et al., 2008).

Yet, there is evidence that feeding has a highly affectionate and social function,[1] as particularly documented from rural contexts in the Global South, such as Papua New Guinea (Barlow, 2001, 2013), Malaysia (Carsten, 1995), Madagascar (Scheidecker, 2025), Micronesia (Quinn, 2013), Mali (True et al., 2001), Indonesia (Seymour, 2013), and India (Chaudhary, 2004). These societies acknowledge the nutritional importance of food, but also stress the interpersonal function of feeding as even more important. For example, in Murik society in Papua New Guinea, children are considered to belong to those who feed them: feeding basically defines belonging, while not being fed implies rejection and separation (Barlow, 2013). In some Asian cultures, kinship is not biologically defined and fixed from birth but develops in the process of being fed and sharing food with others (Carsten, 1995; Janowski & Kerlogue, 2007). For example, Jambi Malays adopting Chinese children believe that they become kin by sharing food (Janowski & Kerlogue, 2007). The cultural value of food and food sharing, also for identity formation ("we are what we eat"), is also reflected in popular cultural-historical documentaries on television, such as "Eating, Power, History", "Kitchen of the World" (ARTE), and "Cultural fights for Food" (3SAT), to name just a few from Germany.

Breastfeeding is part of the sociocultural context of relationship formation. In some cultures, it is considered not only as interpersonal glue, but also as fostering bonds to the community, and thus cultural identity. For example, the Nso believe that breastfeeding symbolically and socially "make someone Nso" (Yovsi & Keller, 2003); even a non-native Nso can become an Nso by being breastfed by an Nso woman. In the Nso and other sub-Saharan cultural communities, this is called milk kinship or fictive kinship.

However, there is also evidence from WEIRD contexts that breastfeeding can be a mechanism through which attachment is formed. Qualitative studies focusing on caregivers' perspectives and attitudes (e.g., using in-depth interviews) repeatedly show that breastfeeding is perceived to be associated with the mother–child attachment. Fostering the mother–child relationship is one of the most important factors reported regarding initiation and continuation of breastfeeding in Dutch families (Gijsbers et al., 2005). The maternal conception of an exclusive, unique attachment relationship with the child through breastfeeding is mentioned in studies from the United States (Wrigley & Hutchinson, 1990), Australia (Schmied & Lupton, 2001), New Zealand (Kronborg et al., 2015), and Spain (Sánchez-Mira & Saura, 2020). Additionally, parenting guides and programs assume a clear association between breastfeeding and the child's attachment to the mother, such as La Leche League International (2020) and attachment parenting (Sears & Sears, 2001), which explicitly or implicitly rest on attachment theory.

In line with qualitative studies conducted in WEIRD (Gijsbers et al., 2005; Kronborg et al., 2015; Sánchez-Mira & Saura, 2020; Schmied & Lupton, 2001; Wrigley & Hutchinson, 1990) and rural contexts of the Global South (Carsten, 1995; Houghtaling et al., 2018; Kerlogue, 2007; True et al., 2001; Scheidecker, 2025; Yovsi & Keller, 2003), breastfeeding mothers regarded breastfeeding as crucial in establishing the early mother–child relationship and for the child's social and emotional development. Breastfed children in middle-class families in San José, Costa Rica, are considered attached, especially to the mother, because she breastfeeds the child.

Yet, breastfeeding is not a causal mechanism. Families in which infants were not breastfed did not report any attachment-related functions of breastfeeding or feeding generally. Even those families who did breastfeed but supplemented with bottle-fed formula milk from early on did not articulate the link between feeding and attachment (Schmidt et al., 2023b). The views of the non-breastfeeding families are thus in line with attachment theory and quantitative studies in WEIRD contexts, stating that feeding is only of limited relevance for the infant–mother attachment (Bowlby, 1958, 1969; Colen & Ramey, 2014; see reviews by Linde et al., 2020; Peñacoba & Catala, 2019).

The findings of the Schmidt et al. (2023b) study further indicate that feeding is perceived as relevant for attachment in a multifaceted and contextualized way depending on the prevalent feeding practices and caregiving setting. The study emphasizes the context specificity of attachment formation. It is in line with evolutionary assumptions that attachment formation should be an environmentally open process, enabling flexibility and adaptability to diverse sociocultural contexts. For example, the reported link between breastfeeding and attachment might be typical for urban middle-class families. Children who are exclusively breastfed by their mothers in rural non-Western families do not seem to form an exclusive attachment to the mother but multiple attachments to several caregivers (Keller, 2007; Yovsi & Keller, 2003). Other mechanisms might come into play to discourage children from forming an exclusive relationship with the mother. For example, in some contexts in India, children are breastfed briefly and intermittently, rarely in a dyadic setting and without much empathic attention (Chaudhary, 2011; Seymour, 2013). The fact that breastfeeding is believed to promote attachment in a population in which attachment theory has assumedly had the greatest influence – namely, the urban middle class (Rosabal-Coto et al., 2017) – is particularly interesting and challenging for attachment theory.

A third entry into the formation of attachment can be ascribed to cultural learning. Suzanne Gaskins et al. (Gaskins et al., 2017) argue that cultural learning shapes how children form attachments by providing the models, routines, and meanings through which infants and caregivers interpret and respond to each other. Cultures differ in norms about caregiver–child interactions (e.g., who is a caregiver, how much physical closeness is needed, what are the channels of communication, and which soothing styles are in place). For example, in some cultures, co-sleeping and close nighttime proximity are normative, with soothing shared among caregivers. Sleep is an affiliative, collective practice. The WEIRD normative view focuses on independent sleeping of infants, alone in a bed/cot or even a separate room from early on. These scripts guide how attachment behaviors are elicited and interpreted. She argues that core needs like safety, comfort, etc., are universal; the culturally learned ways of meeting them vary, leading to attachment styles that are adaptive within a given cultural setting. Bowlby/Ainsworth, on the other hand, focus on the universality of needs for safety and comfort in terms of acquisition and expression.

The cultural learning approach relates to reported specifics of infant–father attachment where play and exploration are considered crucial. However, attachment based on play and exploration is regarded as secondary to meeting the primary needs of closeness (see before).

Gaskins is also concerned about practical applications based on the principle of unconditional universality, like the nurturing care framework (see later), and demands that interventions should be culturally informed, respecting local caregiving norms.

The three entries to the formation of attachment demonstrate that there is not one normative entry that applies to all children and their caregiving environment globally. Three entries are documented in the literature, which were briefly presented here. There may be other entries as well that wait to be documented. It is also obvious that there are context-specific variations, as has been shown with breastfeeding. Presumably, the entries are not distinct categories, but overlap and interact. Further non-confirmatory and contextual research is needed to explore the full spectrum of attachment formation across cultures and contexts.

Note

1 This part is based on Schmidt et al. (2023b).

10

IS ATTACHMENT THEORY A SCIENTIFIC THEORY AT ALL?

Abstract

As a consequence of the previous discussion, the question emerges whether attachment theory is a scientific theory at all. In order to evaluate this question, the usual criteria of a good scientific theory are analyzed against the formulations of attachment theory. The criteria are consistency, testability and falsifiability, predictive power, scope, being based on empirical evidence, ability to evolve, and simplicity. The conclusion is that attachment theory falls short of meeting the criteria for a good theory. The conceptions of attachment theory are often diffuse and unclear (e.g., concerning the definitions of attachment, secure base, internal working model, exploration, sensitivity), partly wrong (e.g., the evolutionary derivation and the assumption of adaptability), and ideologically biased (e.g., the sole consideration of the cultural reality of the Western middle class). Therefore, the name (attachment *theory*) and the common discourse practice need to be revised.

In the following paragraphs, attachment theory will be proved to be a scientific theory. The discussion presented will be structured along the criteria for a good scientific theory.

A good scientific theory has several key characteristics, which are presented below with an assessment of whether attachment theory meets the criteria. The conclusion is that attachment fails in all respects to represent a scientific theory. This has implications for the rationale and justification of applications in many areas of application.

DOI: 10.4324/9781003672050-12

In developmental psychology, a grand theory is considered to

- address development across the lifespan,
- integrate biological, emotional, social, and cognitive aspects
- be applicable across species and cultures,
- have influenced multiple disciplines (e.g., clinical psychology, social work, education, psychiatry).

In this respect, attachment theory would qualify as a grand theory. However, the acceptance of this view depends on the acceptance of the premises. Is it possible at all that a theory not satisfying the criteria listed before can be applicable across cultures? This would necessarily imply an ethnocentric perspective. Researchers based on ethnographic approaches in the study of children's relational development, therefore, come to the conclusion of the inapplicability of attachment theory across cultures (see, e.g., Quinn & Mageo, 2013, Gottlieb, 2004; Otto & Keller, 2014; Keller, 2022a; LeVine et al., 1994).

Based on Empirical Evidence: A scientific theory should be grounded in empirical data obtained through experimentation and observation. It should be supported by a substantial body of evidence.

Attachment researchers would certainly subscribe to the validity of this requirement, pointing to the numerous empirical studies conducted over the last decades. However, most attachment research is restricted methodologically and also conceptually, as has been briefly outlined before. Contemporary attachment researchers, the third generation, themselves also seem to critically question and examine the standard methods, like the Strange Situation Procedure, e.g., with respect to their context-dependence, or to how attachment is expressed in the presence of multiple caretakers, as Robbie Duschinsky (2025) explains with respect to Sheri Madigan's research. However, Madigan is also part of an author collective (Dagan et al., 2021) that claims that in infancy, the gold standard assessment of attachment is an observational paradigm of infant–parent interactions: the Strange Situation Procedure. Madigan is not the only attachment researcher who has stated different opinions within short periods of time. It is not only the differences between different attachment researchers, but also the different positions of the individual attachment researcher, sometimes within the same year, that contribute to the confusion about attachment theory (for example, see Keller, 2022a).[2]

Duschinsky (2025) concludes that attachment research in developmental psychology still remains centered on the child–primary caregiver relationship, with the study of contextual factors acknowledged but not given a central place.

Ability to Evolve: As new evidence emerges, a good theory should be adaptable. Scientists should be willing to revise or refine the theory based on new data without losing its foundational principles.

This has been a problem for a long time, with attachment researchers not being open to adaptability and change in this respect. The research strategy was confirmatory (see before), ignoring and/or minimalizing results that did not fit. For example, the deviations of the attachment classifications from the standard (Baltimore) distribution found by the German attachment pioneers Klaus and Karin Grossmann in their Bielefeld study caused great confusion in the attachment community (see discussion in Karen, 1994). More children were classified as insecure avoidant than had been expected from the norm distribution (Grossmann et al., 1981). It was explained ex post facto as a consequence of a more restricted socialization style forcing the children to immature independence. However, socialization styles or goals were never assessed. The finding was reconciled in the eyes of the attachment community with the replication of the standard distribution in the Regensburg study (Grossmann et al., 1981).

Another deviating distribution resulted from the Sapporo study in Japan. It revealed an unexpectedly high number of insecure ambivalent children, which was later explained by methodological problems in data assessment and analysis. Also, the Kibbutzim studies in Israel reported higher rates of avoidant attachment qualities, which were explained by the communal sleeping arrangements in the kibbutz as disturbing the development of secure attachment relationships (for more details of these studies, see Mesman et al., 2016).

The fundamental interrelationship between culture and attachment was not recognized because findings that were attributed to culture post hoc were regarded as deviations or noise that disturbed the confirmation.

Accordingly, cross-cultural attachment studies used to insist on the strict application of the standard SSP protocol. Numerous inconsistencies in the results were interpreted as not following the standard protocol, training deficiencies, etc. (Mesman, van IJzendoorn and Sagi-Schwartz, 2016). These authors came to the following conclusion in their summary chapter in the *Handbook of Attachment*:

In our chapter of this third edition, which includes attachment data from five new countries or cultures compared to the previous edition (van IJzendoorn & Sagi-Schwartz, 2008), we pay special attention to cross-cultural beliefs about attachment and sensitivity, and we provide more details on attachment and sensitivity in Latin America and with Arabs living in Israel. What has not changed since 2008 is that the available cross-cultural studies have not refuted the bold conjectures of attachment theory about the universality of attachment, the normativity of secure attachment, the link between sensitive caregiving and attachment security, and the competent child outcomes of secure attachment. In fact, taken as a whole, the studies are remarkably consistent with the theory. Until further notice, attachment theory may therefore claim cross-cultural validity (p. 872).

Also, Jude Cassidy comes in the same handbook to an equivalent conclusion: "Bowlby and Ainsworth's original ideas have held up well". And she continues: "... nothing that has emerged from the thousands of studies produced over the past 40 years has led to a serious challenge to the core theory" (Cassidy, 2016, p. 17).

Yet, meanwhile, there are obviously doubts about the validity of those bold statements. In 2021, Judy Mesman concludes: ".... although the conclusion in the chapter on culture in the *Handbook of Attachment*" that "until further notice, attachment theory may... claim cross – cultural validity" (Mesman et al., 2016, p. 809) is attractive, it would be more elegant and productive to rephrase that to say "Until further notice, we need to ask more critical questions before we can firmly claim cross – cultural validity of attachment theory".

A profound and extensive discussion of changes, particularly in the work of the third generation of attachment researchers and the differences between them, is documented by Duschinsky (2025). The third generation asks challenging questions about what elements of attachment research of the prior generations should be preserved, rejected, or renegotiated. Yet the third generation is as heterogeneous as the prior ones; however, Duschinsky has made these differences traceable. He discusses overlapping strata and distinct and semi-competing approaches to attachment research by four groups of third-generation attachment researchers (Duschinsky, 2025). Already their basic conceptualization of constituting terms like attachment security is different. For Lyons-Ruth, security means positive and effective caregiver–child coregulation; for Belsky, security means positive attitudes toward close relationships; for Van IJzendoorn and Bakermans-Kranenburg, security means an individual's feeling of access to a secure base and safe haven provision. Madigan does not seem to have a specific theoretical stake, but regards security as more than the absence of insecurity, like the other groups too. She wants to be clear about what exactly is being measured by various assessments of security, being concerned that these may smuggle in quite various theoretical commitments and have different meanings.

In summary, after a long time during which the attachment community stood firm together as an ingroup, fending off all criticism, a fresh twist seems to acknowledge the need to evolve and the need to take other perspectives into account. Yet the future development will have to show how serious these developments are.

Simplicity: While not a strict rule, simpler theories that explain the same phenomena are generally preferred over more complex ones. Theories should not introduce unnecessary complications.

Attachment theory, on the one hand, is a simple theory if taken the simplistic version that is mostly used. On the other hand, with all the inconsistencies and problems, it is complex and complicated. However, simplicity or parsimony should not override precision and clarity.

In conclusion, the core assumptions and conceptions of attachment theory are far from a sound scientific foundation. They are:

- often diffuse and unclear (e.g., concerning the definition of attachment, secure base, internal working model, exploration, sensitivity).
- partly wrong (e.g., the evolutionary derivation and the assumption of adaptability).
- ideologically biased (e.g., the sole consideration of the cultural reality of the Western middle class).

Thus, attachment theory does not meet the criteria of a good scientific theory. Reliable relationships are important for children to develop trust in others and themselves, thereby opening access to the world. Yet it is not one single model of a dyadic adult (parent/mother) and child relationship that builds security. Jared Diamond (2013) reports with reference to past and traditional societies that responsibility for childcare is diffused among numerous adults and older siblings within the community. This should foster a broader support network and sense of social cohesion, thus providing more stability than the dyadic approach. This diffusion or better network in one or other shape is the prevalent model in many rural communities of the majority world, as has been reported before.

Relational development is not independent of time and space. Declaring one cultural pathway as universal and normative is intrusive and hegemonic. There are obviously different entries to develop significant relationships within and across societies and maybe even cultures, which have been outlined before.

Notes

1 The attachment Q sort is a sorting technique that allows for categorizing descriptive statements about the child regarding attachment-relevant observations.
2 It is not the fact that scientists may not change their views in general. This may be a logical consequence of developments in the field of research. In attachment research, it is puzzling that the same researchers claim continuity and change in the same domain at the same time.

11

CONCLUDING EVALUATION OF ATTACHMENT THEORY

In the previous paragraphs, attachment theory has been critically analyzed with respect to its scientific foundation, its implicit assumptions, and its ethnocentric nature. Cultural anthropologists and cultural psychologists, as well as scientists from other fields, come to the conclusion that attachment theory is a WEIRD conception that does not meet any criterion of a scientifically sound theory (for a summary, see Keller, 2022a).

Although there is now recognition of problems, inconsistencies, and flaws in the circle of attachment researchers, especially the third generation, the theory is still maintained (see Thompson, 2026, Bjorklund, 2026). It is not only regarded as an umbrella for mini attachment theories covering many other topics, as Ross Thompson formulated (2017), but it is also still transmitted and taught in university curricula as well as in applied schools without acknowledging all the reservations and the recognition of problems that attachment researchers themselves admit. The consequence is that a biased, incorrect conception of children's socio-emotional development enters the applied field and serves as the template for different fields of application, irrespective of context and culture.

Attachment theory is considered

> to epitomize the ideal person as emotionally regulated, autonomous yet connected, and capable of healthy intimacy. This is the neoliberal humanist ideal of white fantasy: self-sufficient, rational, and stable.

DOI: 10.4324/9781003672050-13

> Deviation—through culture, oppression, or trauma—is framed as a deficiency, with survival strategies pathologized as disorders.
>
> *(Ayoto, 2025, https://ayoto.substack.com/p/attachment-theory-is-white-supremacy, retrieved 21.1.2026)*

In the following chapter, some of the problems in the applied fields related to child care and parenting will be highlighted. Especially educational practices, parenting interventions in the Global South, as well as the evaluation of parenting in family court decisions are targeted.

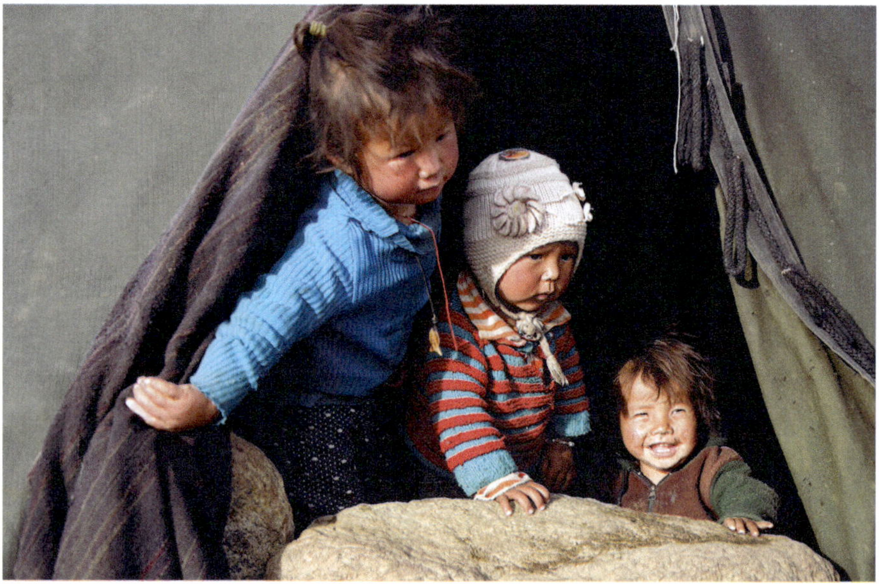

FIGURE 7 Children in Changthang in Laddakh. Copyright Vishwas Raj Adventure Sindbad

PART 3

Attachment and the applied field

More areas of construction

Abstract

Attachment theory is a major player in the applied field. However, the poor empirical basis and the conceptual flaws have not been translated into reservedness toward application. Thus, a bold statement of the assumed scientifically confirmed universal course of early socio-emotional development is reigning the field. Central elements are the exclusive dyadic nature of caregiver–child interactions, the conception of sensitive responsiveness based on eye contact, vocal/verbal responsiveness, and elaboration and stimulation with toys, thus the Bowlby/Ainsworth version of attachment development during the early years. Another building block of application is the classification of attachment qualities and their developmental consequences, thus relying on the competence hypothesis. These assumptions are central in parenting interventions and family court decisions, as well as in early education.

It will be demonstrated that diverse applied fields also follow the same pattern of ignoring the local voices by maintaining the universalistic and normative approach. This is not surprising, since applications are based on so-called scientific evidence, which usually represents the segment of science that follows mainstream rules. But it is more concerning since it interferes directly in people's life with judgments, devaluations, and actions. Three areas will be discussed that are currently more and more debated as pursuing deficiency instead of variability: parenting interventions, family court, custody and child placement, and early pedagogics. Worldwide parenting

DOI: 10.4324/9781003672050-14

interventions as part of Early Child Development programs aim to change socialization styles and parenting, particularly in the Global South, to the WEIRD attachment-based model. This model is also applied in family court decisions, irrespective of the cultural origin of the families. Early pedagogics equally applies attachment-based interactional formats to day care and kindergarten without respecting the possibility that families might have different expectations about early education. The three areas have in common that cultural differences are conceived of as deficiencies that need intervention from outside.

12

PARENTING INTERVENTIONS

Abstract

Parenting interventions generally comprise of all programs directed at supporting children's development through coaching or training parents to improve their parenting. Over the years, parenting interventions have become the center of international aid programs run by global stakeholders like UNICEF, WHO and Non Governmental Organizations (NGO' s). The targets of these programs are mainly families in the global south who are generally evaluated as poor parents based on poverty estimations. Based in attachment theory's conception of sensitive responsiveness, the Nurturing Care Framework has been launched in 2018 by the World Health Assembly. This chapter discusses the scientific and ethical implications of applying one particular conception of parenting to families who follow a completely different socialization agenda. It is argued that the scientific base for these intervention programs ignores the existing research demonstrating the variability of socialization strategies and their benefits in different socio cultural ecologies. It is concluded that parenting interventions often increase structural inequalities.

Parenting interventions generally are structured programs aimed at modifying parental behaviors, skills, and knowledge in order to improve child development and family dynamics.

These interventions range from brief two- to four-session interventions to intensive, multi-month courses. There are different techniques that are used in different programs, such as role-play, video modeling, and live coaching.

DOI: 10.4324/9781003672050-15

Although parenting interventions are in place everywhere, mostly related to counseling and family therapy, such as on an individual basis, the following discussion addresses parenting interventions as part of early childhood development (ECD) interventions in the Global South as a large-scale sector of international development.[1] ECD' philosophy is to improve economic and societal development by impacting young children's development, including their "brain structure and function" (Britto et al., 2017, 97). The need for the improvement is not assessed but is based on estimations of poverty, especially from the estimated number of children who are stunted or live on less than USD 1.90 per day. Thus, it is concluded "that 250 million children (43%) younger than five years in low-income and middle-income countries are at risk of not reaching their developmental potential" (Black et al., 2017, 77). Three Lancet series (for a discussion see Scheidecker et al., 2023) compile what they perceive as scientific evidence about alleged deficits of early child development in the Global South. The assumed deficits of children's development are ascribed to poor parenting ("poor parents parent poorly"). What is understood as quality parenting that is supposed to bring out children's full developmental potential (whatever this means) is what attachment theory proclaims: dyadic parent (mother)-child interactions (although, theoretically, any caregiver can be addressed, mothers are usually targeted, mostly without assessing the factual care arrangements), which follow the patterns described earlier, especially extensive sensitive responsiveness, language use, and stimulation with toys. For example, among seven early learning interventions reviewed by Walker and colleagues in the first Lancet series (2011, 151), six are exclusively directed at mothers while one also includes preschool teachers. On this basis, the WHO, UNICEF, and the World Bank created the Nurturing Care Framework, which was launched in 2018 by the World Health Assembly. Nurturing Care comprises five domains of health, nutrition (which for a long time were the main targets of ECD), security and safety, responsive caregiving, and early learning (Black et al., 2017). Responsive caregiving and early learning are supposed to specifically foster ECD and are therefore prioritized in ECD programs. Britto et al. (2017, 99) claim in one of the Lancet articles that "responsive caregiving" ... "positively affect[s] the child's cognitive and socioemotional development, their brain structure and function, and their physical health". Concerning "early learning", the *Lancet* articles endorse interventions that train caregivers on how to properly play and talk with their children (see Walker et al., 2011, 151). They claim that such parenting interventions improve children's cognitive development, even on the level of "neurocognitive processing and brain functioning" (Engle et al., 2007, 230). The effect of the interventions is ideally measured with randomized controlled trials (RCTs). RCTs are regarded as the gold standard for measuring the effect of interventions by establishing causality. This is believed to be based on minimizing bias and confounding through random assignment to a treatment and a control group. The RCT got momentum with the award of the Nobel Memorial Prize in Economic Sciences to Abhijit Banerjee, Esther Duflo, and Michael Kremer in 2019 for their experimental approach to alleviating global poverty. It is believed that thanks to Abdul Jameel Poverty Action Lab, founded by Banerjee, Duflo, and Sendhil Mullainathan, over 400 million people have been reached by scale-ups of programs that were found to be effective. The main area of ECTs is medical intervention and aid.

However, global medical aid, evaluated with RCTs, can also produce new social disparities in children's lives. Rania Kassab Sweis, an award-winning anthropologist,[2] examines how some of the world's largest aid organizations care for vulnerable children in Egypt, focusing on medical efforts with street children and out-of-school village girls. Ethical issues are obvious with assigning people who need treatment to non-treatment groups. Sweis (2021) argues that millions of dollars are spent each year on global medical aid that often overlooks the local economic and political systems that cause suffering, so that it unintentionally extends the problems.

RCT also found its way into ECD as the gold standard of evaluating interventions. Usually, a group of caregivers (mostly mothers) receiving intervention (attending training sessions on a weekly, bi-weekly, or monthly basis) is compared after some time to a group of mothers not receiving intervention. The content of the training focuses on how to improve the mother–child relationship and to stimulate the child through responsive caretaking and stimulation, usually toy play, in order to enhance the child's cognitive and non-cognitive development. One of the most popular curricula for these types of interventions is the Reach Up and Learn curriculum designed by Grantham-McGregor et al. (2024).

> It is based on the curriculum developed for the Jamaica Home Visiting (JHV) intervention for disadvantaged children up to 4 years of age in LMIC. The JHV curriculum was initially developed in the late 1960s, in response to observations that many children exposed to extreme poverty in Kingston, Jamaica were not reaching their developmental potential. The children lived in unstimulating environments with no toys or books and their mothers had little understanding of the importance of play and responsive interactions.
>
> *(https://doi.org/10.1111/j.1469-8749.1975.tb03527.x)*

The development of a web-based version should enable the transfer to further LMICs, which has meanwhile reached, e.g., Bangladesh, India, Peru, China, and Colombia. Evaluations with RCTs show moderate effects.

In home-based individual or group-based trainings in centers, mothers should learn to

- show consistent love, give positive and specific feedback to the child, and celebrate the child's achievements and efforts.
- observe and being responsive to their child's vocalizations, actions, mood, and interests.

- mediate the environment for the child (drawing attention to, describing, labeling) and introducing new objects, sounds, words, activities, and concepts.
- use play with objects/toys, everyday activities, and looking at books with the child to introduce new concepts and language.

Implementing this parenting style should facilitate children's reaching of their developmental potential (for more details, see https://doi.org/10.1111/j.1469-8749.1975.tb03527.x).

However, despite the achievements of the RCT, debates continue on the role and validity of the RCT method. Some argue that Banerjee, Duflo, and Kremer's success shifts attention and funds away from the big questions, such as how policymakers can tackle the root causes of poverty. Others criticize the RCT method because it makes publishing research more challenging for those who do not use it. And some say that the people doing RCTs have not addressed the issue of agency thoroughly enough in their experiments – if, for example, some groups may be more responsive to intervention than others.

However, the most fundamental criticism addresses the failure to take into account history and context. In parenting intervention evaluations, participants (mothers) in a particular village or area, identified by poverty estimations, are assigned to a treatment or a control group; the history and context of the participant families are seemingly not further considered.

Diamond and Robinson (2010) refer to the important overall issue of ethics. One example is London School of Economics-based Naila Kabeer, who highlights these issues in her research and discusses how the overfocus on RCT methods has led to important findings in relation to gender equality being dismissed (Kabeer, 2024). Diamond and Robinson (2010) opt instead for "natural experiments", which basically means observational studies and ethnographic methodology.

The knowledge base of global ECD is thus questionable with regard to its scientific rigor and, moreover, highly selective and strongly biased. It stems from mainstream research in behavioral sciences like pediatrics, developmental psychology, neurosciences, and behavioral economics and excludes findings from anthropology, cultural psychology, and other relevant fields. There are some studies about populations in the Global South included, which focus on the assessment of supposed deficits as measured by WEIRD standards (Scheidecker et al., 2022; Oppong, 2015). The situation cannot be ascribed to a lack of research. Although non-WEIRD samples are underrepresented in the research landscape, there is nevertheless a substantial body of research that demonstrates the diversity of childrearing models and practices, socialization strategies, and developmental pathways as functions of variable social, cultural, and ecological contexts (for reviews see Keller, 2022a; Lancy, 2022; Rogoff, 2003). So far, however, ethnographic research has been completely ignored in the scientific literature on which global ECD in its current form is based.

Scheidecker et al. (2023) argue that

> The unfortunate situation that highly relevant ethnographic research is de facto irrelevant for global ECD must be ascribed to the disciplinary divides between the fields that produce ethnographic research and the sciences that actually inform child-focused interventions, as others have pointed out (e.g., Hart, 2006; Ochs and Kremer-Sadlik, 2020). Scholars on either side of that divide may be unaware of or reluctant to engage with a body of literature that, although referring to the same subject matter, abides by different scientific procedures, assumptions, and standards.

These authors opt for cross-disciplinary engagement that could also help prevent misguided and potentially harmful interventions and challenge widely publicized claims about "poor" brain development in "poor" countries.

Parenting interventions are not only promoted by the global players like UNICEF or the World Bank but also by numerous Non-Governmental Organizations (NGOs). It is not a surprise that the LEGO Foundation is entertaining a large program of interventions in LMICs with a focus on toy play.

An example of an NGO-based parenting intervention aimed at improving the health and well-being of children and families globally is the "Reinforcement of Parental Practice" (RPP) developed and implemented by the Senegal-based NGO Tostan, supported by the Bill and Melinda Gates Foundation. Tostan aims to "empower African communities to bring about sustainable development and positive social transformation". It started in 2009 and continued in 2022 as the "New RPP" supported by the Bezos Family Foundation. The RPP program is aimed at increasing children's school success by teaching parents to use frequent verbal exchange with their children to provide rich cognitive stimulation, which is critical for brain development. The program also advocates changing "traditional" care practices that may hinder verbal exchanges.

The program covers a teaching part of 48 class sessions and personalized home visits, in which daily interactions are practiced. In the home sessions, mainly mothers are encouraged to use "rich and complex" vocabulary, tell stories, describe objects in detail, and ask questions to help children develop language-processing skills. In interacting play sessions, mothers should learn to copy children's behavior and engage in direct eye contact to build strong emotional and social bonds. The parenting practices are based on attachment-based "positive parenting practices" (Juffer et al., 2023).

The program is applied without any direct proof of the socialization goals, ethnotheories, and caregiving practices in place. This, however, is a crucial necessity, as Oppong and Strader (2022) point out, in order to not disregard or interfere with communities' "ways of living with others" that are ecologically and culturally grounded (Keller & Kärtner, 2013). Thus, the title of the Weber et al. (2017) study is telling: "When cultural norms discourage talking to babies: effectiveness of a parenting program in rural Senegal" (Weber et al., 2017). In rural Senegal, as in many sub-Saharan rural communities, verbal exchanges between children and adults are restricted and repetitive. Children are not supposed to address adults without being asked. Children's answers are expected to be brief, often just assuring what the adult said by saying "yes". Advising mothers to encourage children to use elaborate language is against the social etiquette of the community. There are several studies documenting the communication style of these Senegalese Wolof children (e.g., Rabain-Jamain, 2001) that are not mentioned in the Weber et al. study.

Intending to change cultural practices, such as, reliance on non-verbal communication more than verbalizing, may stigmatize the caregivers who practice them. Changing cultural practices may alter social dynamics and disrupt family or community life, or even increase the likelihood of exposing children to dangers from which they would otherwise be protected by their community's care practices (e.g., Nsamenang, 2007; Serpell & Nsamenang, 2014; see Morelli et al., 2018). In line with the usual practice, the real-world consequences of the program are not studied by Weber et al. (2017).

Ethical principles require respecting people and their values, perspectives, and beliefs, doing no harm, and promoting children's welfare. Encouraging caregivers to radically shift their strategies of care from one kind of care to another represents a sharp discontinuity. Discontinuity in terms of inconsistent parenting is otherwise regarded as a significant risk factor for emotional, social, and cognitive development (e.g., Dollberg & Keren, 2020). Given the claim for universality concerning the application of positive parenting, it is amazing that these claims are neglected or ignored in these cases.

Success in schooling is often regarded as a primary goal of parenting interventions (including the program by Tostan). However, the school discourse in terms of communication style, competitiveness, and individual achievement (see Rogoff, 2003) may undermine the socially responsible intelligence (e.g., respect, obedience, and cooperation) that is expected of children in many rural, subsistence lifestyle communities (e.g., Serpell, 2011). For example, adolescents, who as children dropped out of Western-style primary school and remained in their villages, were rated as less respectful (e.g., Jukes et al., 2018).

One obvious remedy to avoid epistemic violence of this kind is to use ethnographic research. Although the knowledge base is far from complete on a worldwide scale, there is plenty of evidence based on cultural anthropological and psychological ethnographic studies about diversity in the global world. However, ethnographic research has been completely ignored in what is considered the scientific base of global ECD programs (Scheidecker et al., 2023; Morelli et al., 2018).

Change is also needed in the application of codes of ethics. Usually, WEIRD-based researchers act with the approval of the ethics committee of their universities in the Global North. However, these ethical approvals are based on the independent and separate agency of individuals. Trying to act on these premises in the Global South may cause unwarranted consequences for participants in studies, disregarding local norms and values. In our own research program (see Keller, 2022a), we repeatedly faced awkward situations; e.g., Indian lower-middle-class participants felt distrust on our part when asked to sign informed consent forms. For them, verbal agreement was the way to go. Rural Indian village heads of families did not let us have young mothers sign consent forms, since the household head was in change of granting permission or not. In retrospect, we realized that we not only violated local forms of conduct but also put the young mothers in a painful situation. In Nso villages in the Northwest of Cameroon, we had to seek the approval of the local king (Fon) in order to address families. An impressive example is what a Costa Rican anthropologist told about working with an indigenous group in Costa Rica, which sent a delegation to the university to protest against the granted anonymity in the consent agreement because they insisted that their names were explicitly mentioned.

These are just a couple of examples underlining that consulting ethnographic research is mandatory for researchers from the Global North, but that it is even more important, to design research projects cooperatively with locals on an equal basis.

There are some local ethical codes, like "the African Charter on the Welfare and Rights of the Child" from the Organization of African Unity (https://resourcecentre.savethechildren.net/document/african-charter-rights-child).

This code stresses local values by stating in the preamble "the virtues of their cultural heritage, historical background, and the values of the African civilization".

Article II specifies that the child's education should include "the preservation and strengthening of positive African morals, traditional values and cultures". There are also codes of ethics from the San of South Africa, the First Nations in Canada, the Aboriginal and Torres Strait Islanders in Australia, and the New Zealand Maori Guidelines. They all stress the need to consult with local communities first, community control, collective decision-making, and benefit-sharing (for more discussion, see also Morelli et al., 2018).

Researchers working in the Global South often must adhere to the Global Code of Conduct for Research in Resource-Poor Settings, which requires showing respect for local ethics committees and obtaining community assent before beginning work.

The problems go even deeper when structural reasons are turned into individual shortcomings. As outlined before, parenting interventions aim to impose WEIRD parenting strategies onto rural families in the Global South. Ongoing parental undivided attention to an individual child, however, clashes with the demands of a rural lifestyle, where children, household, farming/trading, and many other responsibilities have to be attended to at the same time, and care is located in the group. Thus, the intervention programs demand the impossible and may create guilt among mothers. Such structural inequalities are relocated to the level of individual mothers' parenting behavior. Besides all the scientific problems inherent in attachment theory, parenting interventions of this kind must be regarded as acts of epistemic violence and ethical transgressions.

Notes

1 This discussion is partly based on Scheidecker et al. (2023).
2 Book Prize from the Association for Middle East Childhood and Youth Studies for her book, *Paradoxes of Care: Children and Global Medical Aid in Egypt*.

13

FAMILY COURT DECISIONS AND CHILD CUSTODY

Abstract

Family Court decisions concerning child custody should be based in the best interest of the child. However the UN Convention of the Rights of the Child is based in Western middle class ideas about childhood and parenting. Accordingly, often children from families with a migration or refugee background become targets of child welfare systems and family courts in the global north. Two family histories are presented, the path of suffering of an Indian family in Norway and the still ongoing nightmare of an Indian family in Germany. In both cases state authorities ignored children' s rights to grow up in their culture, language, religion, but claimed to act in the children' s best interest. Both cases are also exemplar to demonstrate the misuse of attachment theory. Leading attachment researchers more and more raise their voices to warn of this inherently wrong understanding of attachment theory like e.g. the application of a group based research instrument to individual diagnoses, notwithstanding its application to families with different child care philosophies.

Another applied area, where decolonization is urgently needed, is the family court and especially child placement and custody decisions. The child's best interest (see UN Convention on the Rights of the Child (UNCRC; UN General Assembly 1989)) has become the standard of evaluation. However, the notion of the best interest of the child is a vague concept that needs further specification. This is how attachment theory came into play in defining a supportive environment for children's development and well-being (see Forslund et al., 2021). Attachment and attachment qualities are referenced in

DOI: 10.4324/9781003672050-16

evaluations concerning custody and child placement decisions. That means that the diversity of child-rearing ideas and practices is evaluated along one conception of parenting quality, i.e., the universal and normative assumptions of attachment theory.

Especially families and single mothers with a migration or refugee background are, thus, targeted for unresponsive parenting. Amici et al. (2026) examined possible biases in social interventions regarding children from different cultural backgrounds. They conclude based on statistics from many WEIRD countries that "the data show a highly consistent trend across countries: children from minority cultural backgrounds are disproportionately represented in child protection systems".

An example is the sad story of the Indian Bhattacharya family in Norway that received worldwide attention. Mr. Bhattacharya moved from India to Norway to accept a job as an IT specialist in an oil company. After living and working for one year in Norway, he decided that he would like to marry and found a family. In order to find a wife, he traveled back to India because he wanted to marry an Indian woman. Mr. Bhattacharya married a young woman from South India who followed him to Norway, her first trip away from home and abroad. The young family soon had two children and tried to settle in Norway. The young woman, however, did not feel comfortable without any relatives and friends in a foreign country. The marriage did not go as smoothly as expected. Mrs. Bhattacharya felt completely overstrained with a household in a strange environment, a husband who was mostly absent because of his work obligations, two small children – and all this without the support of her extended family. The then two-year-old son went to a local kindergarten where the teachers noticed behavioral problems. They informed the responsible institution, the Norwegian Child Welfare Service (CWS, Barnevernet). Staff members visited the family at home, observing and videotaping. After a couple of visits during the following months, they decided to take both children into out-of-home care because Mrs. Bhattacharya did not conform to the ideas of a caring and responsible mother that they had. There was no communication about educational ideas between the CWS and the mother because the staff members did not speak Tamil, a South Indian language, and the mother did not speak Norwegian. The two-year-old son and the then five-month-old daughter were submitted to state custody and placed in foster families. This decision came as a complete surprise to the parents. After a battle lasting many years with the Norwegian authorities, and only after the intervention of the Indian government, the children were transferred to India, but to the paternal family. However, the couple was separated in the meantime and divorced eventually. But Mrs. Bhattacharya did not stop fighting until she was assigned the sole custody of her children. Today she lives with her children in Kolkata and works as a software development engineer (see also www.masalachaimusings.com). The Indian lawyer, artist, and child activist Suranya Aiyar (saveyourchildren.in) supported her tremendously. Sagarika Chakraborty's (Mrs. Bhattacharya's maiden name, which she took on again after divorce) life took a substantial turn. She studied and wrote a book about the nightmare she had gone through: "The Journey of a Mother" (Vishwakarma Publications, 2022). The film director Nikkhil Advani released, in 2023, a Hindi (Bollywood) film, based on Sagarika's book: Mrs. Chatterjee vs Norway. The movie received worldwide attention, much to the dismay of the Norwegian government.

What were the reasons for the Norwegian Child Welfare Service to take the children out of their family? The mother seemed to be overstrained and exhausted; she barely had eye contact with the baby, did not react sensitively, did not talk much to the children, and raised her hand toward the boy, which was seen as being close to beating, but in fact represents a gesture of setting limits in many Indian regions. The Norwegian staff evaluated the behavior they had observed according to attachment theory. They did not deal with the mother's ideas, intentions, or attitudes. Of course, the mother was overstrained, also because of the home visits of the Welfare Service, which she did not understand. Why were these people coming, spending time in her house, taking notes? The mother was certainly in need of support to cope with her problems in a foreign country, her loneliness, and her disappointment with her marriage. Nobody in this whole process ever took notice of her as a human being. And obviously, nobody cared about what the disaster of taking away the children would cause to the mother, the children, and the dynamics of the whole family. And how can anybody think that this is in the best interest of children?

Another telling story is that of the Indian girl Ariha Shah, who came under the control of the German Youth Office (Jugendamt). Her sad story is partly documented in a paper by Prayathna Kowitz addressing the cultural and human rights ignorance of institutions in the Global North when the best interest of a child, particularly from a family originating in the Global South, is defined (Kowitz, 2023). The publication of the real name and thus the identity of the child and the family is fully consented to by the parents. The Indian Jain family Shah moved from Gujarat, India, to Berlin due to the father's professional employment. Her first child, Ariha, was born in Berlin and has an Indian passport. In September 2021, the parents took their then seven-month-old girl to a pediatrician because they had noticed bleeding in her diaper. Following check-ups in a hospital, it was stated as "hormonal bleeding". A couple of days later, a new doctor in the hospital got suspicious during a voluntary follow-up check-up about possible child abuse.

Due to COVID restrictions at that time, the mother, who did not speak German, was alone with Ariha in the hospital. She did not understand what was going on and signed all documents that were handed to her in order to provide the best treatment for her daughter. The Youth Office was called in, and Ariha was transferred from the hospital to a temporary foster home. The shocked parents were asking for the medical files, which they received only after several requests over months. The parents insist to this day that they do not know how the injury could have happened. However, the paternal grandmother, who visited the family at that time, confessed that she had accidentally hurt the girl during diaper changing. Yet she never came under allegation. With the help of the Indian lawyer and child activist Suranya Aiyar, the family solicited numerous evaluations of the documents by external medical doctors. Although all charges against the parents were dropped, including allegations of sexual abuse, Ariha became a civil case for custody in the family court.

Two years later, Ariha was placed without prior announcement in institutional care because the foster parent retired (which was well known ahead of time to the institution, but not to the family). For Ariha, this meant another abrupt change in her life. The parents were allowed a monthly and later bi-monthly one-hour visit. Nevertheless, Ariha maintained a bond with her parents, which was, amazingly enough, the reason for being diagnosed as disorganizedly attached. This led to Ariha's placement into a unit for children with special needs.

Ariha was systematically alienated from her cultural roots by the German authorities. All requests for contact with Gujarati, the native language of the Shahs were refused. The Shah family lives according to the Jain rules of life, which means, e.g., strict dietary commandments, including absolute non-violence (Ahimsa), aimed at causing the minimum possible harm to any living being. It restricts all meats, eggs, and root vegetables, prohibits eating after sunset, and requires carefully filtered water. The Jain population worldwide that raises their children according to their dietary rules comprises more than 6 million people. However, it was devalued as not being in according with the WHO guidelines and as constituting a "health hazard" for a small child. The treatment of Ariha clearly contradicts the Universal Declaration of Human Rights and the UN Convention on the Rights of the Child, which clearly state that every child has the right to live their own culture, to practice their own religion, and to use their own language. This right explicitly also applies to children who are temporarily or permanently deprived of their family environment. The interventions of the Indian embassy were not considered.

Meanwhile, Ariha is almost five years of age and has lived with four foster families over time. The parents are allowed to see her every two weeks. Despite the long time with varying time spans of contact deprivation, Ariha has remained attached to her parents and keeps asking them why she cannot go home with them. She seems to resignate and announced that when she is an adult and decides herself about her stay she will move (back) to her parents. There was some political action, also involving the foreign ministry that led to an agreement that Ariha should be in touch with Gujarati or at least Hindi and be in contact with an Indian community. However, nothing has worked out.

Ariha's sad story demonstrates again that the best interest of a child is often an arena for manipulation in the service of power. The principle of the child's best interest is used to assert that the Youth Office is the only authority that decides who raises a child taken out of a family and where. With the abrupt changes of caregivers and locations, the authorities are violating their own principle that changes are situations of crisis that need to be specifically staged in order to avoid harm to the child (as can be seen, e.g., in regulations regarding the transition from home to institutional care like day care or kindergarten).

These are not single cases. Plenty of sad stories are documented worldwide. Cultural modes of parenting are evaluated against attachment assumptions/prescriptions and a priori evaluated as a deficit. Experts who are assessing the family relationships and the child's situation are often biased. They often do not explore the family's realities but take bits and pieces selectively to validate their opinion. This is the same confirmatory method that has characterized attachment theory and research for a long time.

Plenty of information is available describing and explaining cultural differences in parenting and socialization strategies, which experts do not know about or ignore. If there is an awareness of other beliefs and practices, the reaction often is: "Ok, in their home place they may do it this way, but now they are here, and have to do it our way". This is, of course, an indefensible attitude, not only ethically. It has been demonstrated with Latino migrants in the USA that maintaining the family values and the mother tongue are, in fact, protecting factors, facilitating integration (Marks & Garcia-Coll, 2012).

Irish children's rights activist Joe Burns has made the point by saying that in thousands of years of human history, the family has become the ultimate child protection system in all cultures. The vast majority of children all over the planet are well cared for by their families and communities. Burns also says that the state is the worst possible protector of children, especially in the Western world. He refers to analyses of economist Joseph Doyle Jr. (2007), who had demonstrated that children who get into the purview of state officers, who have higher records of taking children out of their families, are probably also placed in foster families. They have later higher crime rates, teenage pregnancies, and lower economic security than children who remain in their families, even if these families are regarded as difficult. Although the relationships were statistically weak, the tendency was nevertheless clear. There are, of course, cases where intervention is necessary, but the number of false positives by far exceeds the number of children at real risk.

The problematic application of attachment theory to family court decisions is also recognized by attachment researchers. 70 of the internationally leading attachment researchers from 23 countries have published in 2021 a consensus article with the title: "Attachment goes to court: child protection and custody issues" (Forslund et al., 2021), in which they express their concerns about how attachment theory is (mis)used in family court decisions. They argue that

> Accurate implementation of attachment theory and attachment assessments in this context has, however, been hampered by a variety of factors. First, there is a great deal of misinformation about attachment in circulation across various contexts, including the family courts. This includes misinformation about fundamental matters such as what attachment is, the nature of children's multiple attachment relationships, and what can be inferred – at the level of an individual child – from assessments of attachment quality (Granqvist et al., 2017).
>
> *(Forslund et al., 2021, p. 7)*

One of the main problems is the reference to attachment qualities for decisions about individual children. Forslund et al. (2021, p. 15) argue that

> Measures to assess attachment quality, when used by trained and certified coders in validated settings, are impressive tools for research on the *group-level.* Yet, questions arise regarding the transferability of the measures' validity to family court settings and *individual* children (and caregivers).

Wrongly generalizing relationships observed at the group level to the individual level is called the ecological fallacy (see Thorndike, 1939; Robinson, 1950).

Moreover,

> …the effect sizes for the associations among children's attachment quality, pertinent caregiving behaviour, and subsequent child development are small to moderate. Consequently, attachment measures do not have sufficient predictive power to serve as stand-alone "proxies" for individual children's caregiving history or how they will develop.
>
> *(Forslund et al., 2021, p. 15)*

Peer Granquist, one of the authors of the Forslund et al. paper, comments on the continuation of an undue practice in the social services in general in an interview with the Swedish journalist Christian Dahlström: "It is really strange that it just continues. It's as if social services live their own life in this area", he says. He describes the practice "to lift uncertain group results out of their research context and translate them to the individual level in order to make life-determining decisions about small children's futures as "catastrophic"" (Interview in Kvatal, "Anknytningsteorin och makten över barnen", February 5 2026).

Forslund et al. (2021) acknowledge

> ...that the community of attachment researchers, including many of us, have at times inadvertently contributed to this situation (Duschinsky, 2020). We have occasionally advocated our methods to assess attachment quality and exaggerated the implications of pertinent findings without explicitly acknowledging their constraints and limitations. In hindsight, it is plain to see that we should have been more careful.
>
> *(p. 15)*

Thus, family court decisions concerning custody and child placement urgently need a complete change of perspective to meet the acclaimed standards of the child's best interests.

14

EARLY PEDAGOGICS

Abstract

Early pedagogics follow the same universal and normative stance than the other applied areas, briefly portrayed before. It is assumed that education and learning are based in attachment relationships. Felt security in relationships is assumed to enable children to explore the environment, and to assess and process information. Learning thus is conceived of as an individual process of an individual child. Documented cultural and interindividual differences in perception and learning styles are not taken into consideration for curricula development. Many children, however, acquire and process information easier in communal and contextualized processes. Alternative learning models as e.g. "learning through observation and pitching in" are presented. Disparities in educational success could probably be minimized by introducing diversity and variability in education and pedagogics.

Also, early education is modeled worldwide along WEIRD conceptions of teaching and learning, although cultural styles of perception, information acquisition and processing, as well as teaching styles, have been documented for quite some time. Most prominent is, e.g., the differentiation into analytic and holistic cognitive styles that manifest in how individuals distribute attention, categorize objects, and attribute causality. The analytic style is more common in WEIRD environments and thus prevalent in school curricula. It focuses on focal objects independent of their context and prioritizes categorization based on formal rules and attributes. More popular in many parts of the world is the holistic style emphasizing the entire field and the relationships

DOI: 10.4324/9781003672050-17

between objects and their background (Nisbett, 2019). These styles not only characterize cultural priorities, but also interindividual preferences, emerging early in life (see, e.g., Varnum et al., 2010). Thus, teaching in one style necessarily disadvantages children who prefer another style. Different styles can be primed and/or learned. However, learning psychologists have argued for a long time that children learn best when they can connect to prior knowledge and routines. The German learning psychologist Elsbeth Stern (2023), e.g., argues that children do not learn from a blank slate; they use existing "schemata" (mental frameworks) to filter and organize new information.

Attachment theory-based conceptions of learning and teaching dominate early education settings like day care and kindergarten. It is taken for granted that educational processes are located in adult–child interaction, expressed in the teacher–child ratio as the non plus ultra of pedagogical quality, face-to-face contact, the importance of language and verbal expressiveness, child-centeredness, and toy stimulation. The credo is that education is not possible without attachment. This signifies, on the one hand, that a secure attachment to the primary caregiver enables the child to explore the world and learn. On the other hand, it also includes that a secure relationship with the kindergarten teacher is a prerequisite for learning (see Keller, 2022a, for more details).

An example of a different learning model is Barbara Rogoff's LOPI model, "Learning by Observation and Pitching In". The basic assumptions of the model are:

Inclusion: Children are integrated into mature community activities rather than being segregated in specialized child-only environments.

Initiative: Children contribute voluntarily for the sake of the collective, often "pitching in" without being asked.

Collaborative Interaction: Participants coordinate their actions fluidly as an ensemble, often using both verbal and nonverbal communication.

Transformation of Participation: Learning is viewed as a process of changing one's role and responsibility within a community, rather than just acquiring bits of information.

Keen Observation: Learners pay wide, broad attention to ongoing activities to understand how to contribute effectively.

Barbara Rogoff (e.g., Rogoff & Mejía-Arauz, 2022) developed this model primarily through ethnographic research in Indigenous-heritage communities of the Americas, such as Mayan communities in Guatemala. In these and many other rural communities of the Global South, learning is a group activity and builds on processes that naturally occur in groups, like observing what others are doing and imitating it. Such learning is deeply contextualized in processes and functions. Children see what learning is for and what the result is.

Rogoff contrasts LOPI with "Assembly-Line Instruction", the dominant model in Western schools where learning is managed by adults in isolated steps in a separate environment. Learning is decontextualized and addresses the universal child individually. Yet, individualization does not refer to the history and learning style of the child, but rather tries to realize uniform pedagogical quality. There is one interesting twist with the conception of "playful learning", which is widely discussed in early pedagogies. It means to present learning topics in a playful manner, as a game. This implies developing a story around the learning topic, which is nothing but contextualizing. However, in line with the dominant conception of childhood, it is not the real world that comes into play, but a simulation designed to make it "child appropriate".

Marie Battiste (2017) documents the nature of Eurocentric models of education in relation to Indigenous knowledge systems. She understands the educational system as forced assimilation and, thus, an act of colonization. She proposes a new model of education that incorporates both Indigenous and Eurocentric thinking (see also Lopez & Singh, 2024; Barongo-Muweke, 2016). There is generally more emphasis on Indigenous learning with a focus on "Indigenous control of Indigenous education" in the Global South. The 2026 Assembly of First Nations Education Forum highlights the integration of Indigenous languages and lifelong learning as vital tools for cultural resurgence.

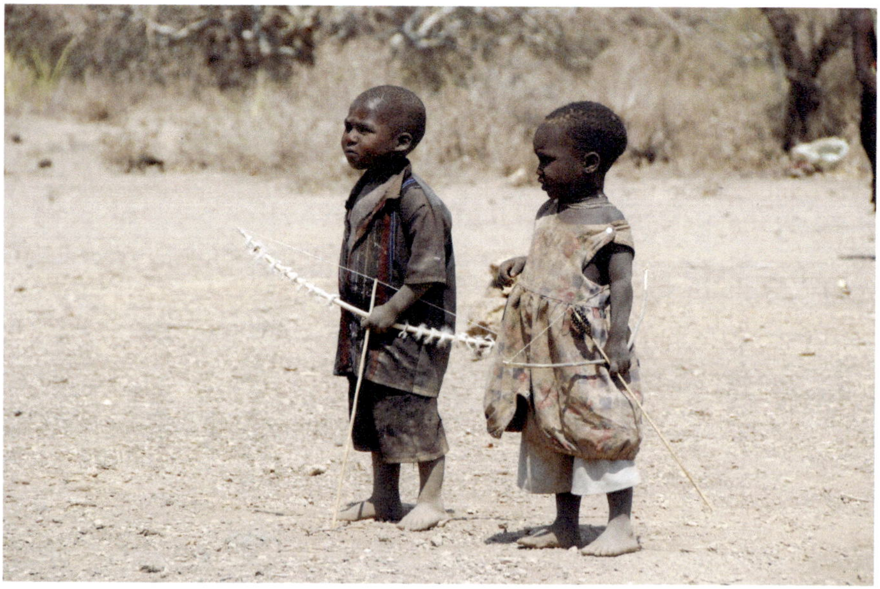

FIGURE 8 Hadzabe children close to Lake Eyasi in Tanzania. Copyright Kristin Moritz

In general, there is meanwhile a remarkable movement that aims to decolonize education as an ongoing process of dismantling Eurocentric dominance in knowledge systems and rebuilding educational structures to honor diverse, global, and Indigenous perspectives that focus on epistemic justice and restorative futures.

In a world where global asymmetries and epistemic injustice have become unmistakably visible, critical reflection on knowledge hierarchies has become increasingly urgent. The Decolonization Forum 2026: Decolonizing Knowledge Production and Circulation aims to bring together scholars, researchers, and intellectuals from around the world to critically examine dominant paradigms, share alternative frameworks rooted in local and Indigenous knowledge, and envision decolonial futures across disciplines (decolonizationforum.org, retrieved 15.1.2026).

Disparities in educational chances are widely discussed in the Western world. There is an awareness that equal opportunities are key to educational achievements. However, the reasons for the status quo are not spotted in different starting positions of children's information acquisition and processing styles. Decolonizing education would thus lead to eliminating bias and truly offering equal access to education. As Doris Bischof-Köhler emphasized many years ago with respect to gender differences, equal treatment of boys and girls does not necessarily lead to equality of outcomes, because their behavioral differences are partly rooted in biology and not solely in socialization (Bischof-Köhler, 2011). Thus, facilitating equal chances may imply different treatment.

3.1 Conclusion

The three applied areas, which are discussed here, have in common that WEIRD attachment-based ideas and behaviors are considered universally valid and, moreover, qualitatively superior to local practices. They address the caregiver/parent as well as the child. They are believed to bring out children's full developmental potential (parenting interventions), set the stage for early learning and education (early pedagogics), and serve children's best interests for security and well-being (custody and child placement). In fact, they are examples of WEIRD hegemonic thinking and epistemic violence as outlined before.

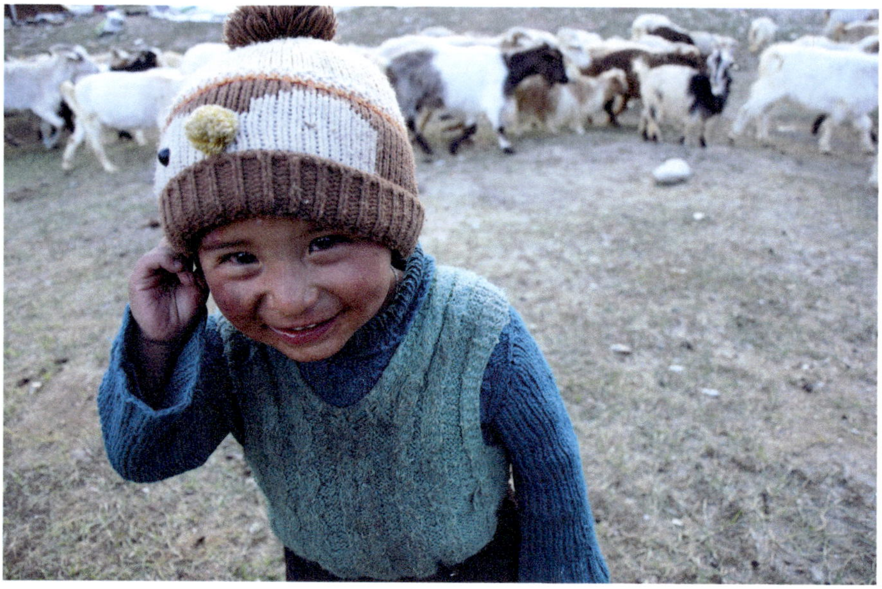

FIGURE 9 Child in Changthang in Laddakh. Copyright Vishwas Raj Adventure Sindbad

PART 4
Problems of change

Abstract

Although there is widespread criticism and concern, within and outside attachment theory, in the Global South as well as the Global North, mainstream views still remain dominant. Why is change not occurring? There are different possibilities that may explain ignorance and resistance. One possibility is structural reasons of power and control, which are located in the WEIRD world and are not abandoned. The other possibilities are psychological issues of maintaining one's own worldview and presumptions considered superior. These presumptions may operate consciously or nonconsciously. Finally, a stairway to change is proposed with four steps to more diverse and inclusive science.

DOI: 10.4324/9781003672050-18

15

IGNORANCE AND RESISTANCE

Abstract

This chapter discusses possible reasons of resistance to change despite growing evidence of ethnocentric and colonial attitudes and practices in science and application. Two complex sets of reasons are offered, one more political and one more psychological. Political reasons may comprise of control and privilege related issues pertaining to the concentration of power and resources in the global north. However, researchers from the global south obviously also help to maintain the status quo by academic allyship, which may relate to perceived career opportunities. Psychological reasons may pertain to explicit and implicit assumptions based in world-views taken as universal truth. For psychology, particularly, the physics envy may represent the desire to be recognized as a hard science, based in quantitative methodology and producing universal truths. More openness and collaboration with anthropology and ethnographic methodology is necessary for promoting inclusiveness.

As outlined in the previous chapters, there is massive scientific and ethical critique concerning WEIRD psychology in general and attachment theory in particular. It has also become clear that a large portion of scientific evidence is ignored and excluded from the mainstream knowledge base. Over the last few decades, many scholars from the Global South as well as from the Global North have raised their voices to dismantle power structures and politics in science. Concepts like colonization, epistemic violence, and ethnocentrism have become central in this discussion. There are many papers and also books available by now, e.g. Tuli and Chaudhary (2025), Tuli and Negi (2025),

DOI: 10.4324/9781003672050-19

Bhatia, Fernández, and Sonn (2025), Smith (1999), and Sanches de Oliveira and Baggs (2023), to name just a few. However, this critique is not new and does not represent a new awareness. Toomela and Valsiner (2010) argue that new developments are seemingly historically blind. They conclude from the chapters of their edited book that 60 years of psychology have gone astray. They think that to go 60–70 years back "a true goldmine of brilliant ideas would open for psychologists" (p. xii).

The question that necessarily arises is why brilliant ideas were not pursued further or did not find their way into the mainstream. Why are brilliant ideas abandoned?

In a commentary on the target article of Bard, Keller, and Leavens (2026) in BBS, Syed (2026) is most explicit in answering this question: "The reality is that psychology wants to stay WEIRD, not go WILD". WILD is an acronym for Worldwide, In Situ, Local, Diverse that was coined by Newson et al. (2021). Bard et al. vote for going WILD in order to make psychological theories and research more diverse and inclusive. Already in 2007, Branco acknowledged "resistance to change (,) on the part of psychological research…" (p. 42).

Yet, why does psychology want to stay WEIRD? There are two complex patterns of reasons possible, one political and one psychological.

The political complex of reasons includes privilege, power, and control. The concentration of research power in the Global North is inextricably linked to historical and ongoing geopolitical structures. The Majority World regions are often situated within a history of colonialism and neo-imperialism. This has created long-term economic and social inequalities that limit the development of independent research infrastructures in these regions.

Thus, WEIRD researchers usually possess and control the resources in terms of funding, institutional support, and publishing possibilities. Research money, fellowships, etc. usually come from institutions and funding agencies in the Global North, which are regarded as more reliable in managing resources. Institutions in the Global North are usually better equipped with staff and administrative facilities. The high-ranked journals are published in the Global North, and the majority of reviewers and editors also come from the Global North.

However, researchers from the Global South also contributed to maintaining the power structures through epistemic allyship, as the late Seth Oppong (2023) named it (see also Scheidecker et al., 2023). Majority world researchers may follow the WEIRD agenda for a variety of reasons, including (1) they have been taught to do so at university; (2) doing so demonstrates their competence and professional authority; and (3) to have access to publication opportunities, research funding, career chances, etc. Nevertheless, the main responsibility for redistributing epistemic authority is in the Global North. This also addresses the question of cooperation. Usually, the Principal Investigators in research studies are identical to the receivers of the funding, i.e., the scholars from the Global North. In order to induce change, collaboration on equal terms is mandatory. Among many others, Seth Oppong advocated strongly for bidirectional relationships in collaborations between academics from the majority world and influential scholars in the minority world who "genuinely want to see another human progress rather than seeing the one in need of assistance as merely a member of a marginalized group" (Oppong, 2023, p. 76). There is also a strong group at Delhi University, India, whose voices are also heard in the scientific community (e.g., Tuli & Chaudhary, 2025). Although there seems to be a broad awareness, change remains slow.

The second complex of hindrances for change concerns psychological reasons, mainly those of the scientists themselves. Most researchers are trained in WEIRD universities and are from WEIRD backgrounds. They tend to take their worldview for granted as a universal truth (see the assumption of universality). Stephen Gould (1996, p. 57) has expressed explicitly that "the most erroneous stories are those we think we know best – and therefore never scrutinize or question".

The worldview influences the types of questions researchers ask and the methodologies they use. These choices, processes, and decisions may go unnoticed since researchers are identified with their own cultural worldview. The conception of the separate, psychological, autonomous agent directs attention to particular questions and problems and overshadows others. Frans de Waal, e.g., demonstrated with his research on non-human primates that Japanese researchers primarily studied cooperation, whereas Euro-American researchers were primarily interested in conflict and competition (de Waal, 2001). In order to change, researchers would need to question their own perspectives and be curious about others. Syed (2026) argues that

> From its early days, psychology revealed an interest in becoming a discipline that generates universal claims about behavior and mental processes. As the field came of age towards the middle of the 20th century, it committed to modeling itself after the natural sciences, in which legitimate knowledge was defined as quantitative in nature and universal.

The model that psychology tries to imitate is physics, as Norbert Bischof argued in 1981 in a programmatic talk at Zurich University. Physics is a fundamental science aimed at finding universal laws, which operates deterministically, ahistorically, and irrespective of context. Bischof argued that physics is the wrong model for psychology. He suggested biology as the better choice since psychological phenomena are like biological systems, complex, historical, and goal-oriented. Also, Syed (2026) confirms that psychologists have physics envy. Mainstream psychology accordingly is based on "hard data", quantitatively oriented with theory-driven experiments as the method of choice. Branco (2007) observes that researchers cling to a positivist approach because they fear losing the status of presenting reliable data, as most typical hard sciences usually do. He observes that "researchers in psychology still feel much more comfortable with the pseudo "objectivity" of their data when facing the broader community of scientists" (p. 43).

Ethnographic qualitative and context-conscious methods are considered unscientific. Accordingly, they are not included in the curricula of universities and training institutions. However, there is an increasing number of cultural psychologists and cultural anthropologists who argue for the necessity to cooperate (see, e.g., Scheidecker et al., 2023). For future progress in going WILD, closer cooperation of anthropologists, psychologists, and other disciplines is mandatory (see also Bard et al., 2026). Obviously, psychology has a serious identity crisis without recognizing it.

Hopefully, the combined forces of anthropologists and psychologists will help to increase the visibility of cultural psychology and to end its existence as a "second psychology" (Cahan & White, 1992). This also includes that cultural/cross-cultural studies are not restricted to journals devoted to culture but enter mainstream publication outlets (Cheung, 2012).

In the applied field, the resistance to change paradigms and methodology is even more pressing, since it directly affects large parts of the world population through, e.g., parenting interventions, custody decisions, and educational philosophies. Seye Abimbola and colleagues (2024) describe convincingly the resistance to change related to an intervention aimed at improving childbirth outcomes in Uttar Pradesh, India, funded by the Bill and Melinda Gates Foundation. The intervention consisted of an eight-month coaching-based implementation of the Safe Childbirth Checklist. Semrau et al. (2017, 2020) tested, among other things, the effect in a randomized controlled trial on a composite outcome of perinatal death, maternal death, or maternal severe complications eight to 42 days after delivery in the intervention group and a control group adjusted for clustering and matching. The results revealed that there was no significant difference in the combined maternal death, neonatal death, stillbirth, and maternal severe complications within seven days after delivery between the intervention facilities and the control. Thus, obviously, the intervention had no effect. Yet the authors (Semrau et al., 2017) did not take the evidence seriously when they conclude:

> One potential interpretation of our findings is that increasing adherence to these practices is not a worthwhile goal, because these practices did not lead to improved outcomes. We strongly believe this conclusion to be false. Each of the practices incorporated in the checklist has its own evidence base, including effectiveness with regard to improving maternal outcomes, improving neonatal outcomes, or both. Evidence of the benefits

> of proper hand hygiene for labouring women and their children, for example, dates back to the 1800s.
>
> *(p. 237)*

Abimbola et al. (2024, pp. 240, 241) discuss two hypotheses addressing this factual ignorance.

The first hypothesis is that perhaps they knew about contextual conditions and peculiarities but did not want to accept their influence. They possibly wanted a simple solution that is not dependent on context and therefore ignored the results.

> They chose, it seems, to be unaware of the temporal context even though they had a good enough sense of how things may evolve over time – in the intervention and in the location. That is, their unawareness may be motivated, a related unawareness, or what we do not (want to) know.
>
> *(Abimbola et al., 2024, p. 241)*

Referring to what Linsey McGoey called "strategic unknowns" (McGoey, 2012) or "strategic ignorance" (McGoey, 2019), they name it "motivated unawareness".

The second hypothesis they present is genuine unawareness, meaning that the authors truly did not know. This hypothesis comes close to what we have discussed as structural reasons before, like

> the tunnel vision that comes with academic discipline, with how academic training disciplines our minds to see the world .... The tunnel vision may be the result of how the authors were educated to become practitioners of public health and medicine, or how they were educated in their quest to become elite researchers with academic careers.
>
> *(Abimbola et al., 2024, p. 241)*

This applies to psychologists and many other social sciences as well. Levins and Lewontin (1985) speak of "specialized education", expressing that education is not restricted to the curriculum but also carries a worldview.

Abimbola and colleagues (2024) give further examples from the structural domain when they claim that high-ranked journals would probably not publish a study in the service of change and that well-known foundations would likely not fund studies focusing on system change. We (leadership by Nandita Chaudhary, Gabriel Scheidecker, and the late Seth Oppong) had similar experiences with the German-based Strüngmann Forum a couple of years ago, which cancelled an already approved Forum on the scientific bases of early childhood development (ECD) and parenting intervention because they found at some very late point the applicants too one-sided, although there was a substantial number of traditional ECD-conform scholars on the invitees' list.

Science seems to be a marketing strategy. Just as vacuum cleaners or vitamin pills are sold better with scientific backup, attachment theory, parenting interventions, and school curricula are sold with so-called scientific evidence. Even if people do not believe the validity of this science, they nevertheless buy the products, as marketing research has proved.

Thus, there is a long way to go. The structural and psychological reasons keep each other mutually alive. But the increasing number of scholars worldwide gives hope that science, at some point, hopefully not too far away, will keep up to its standards.

16

THE STAIRWAY TO CHANGE

Abstract

Based on Bard, Keller & Leavens' (2026) proposal of five steps to change, a modified four step version is proposed. Step 1 comprises of a substantial contextual assessment of the phenomenon under study. Besides scrutinizing existing ethnographic evidence, observational and interview methodology should be employed. Interpretation needs to be based in local knowledge systems. Step 2 addresses the developmental context of the phenomenon, the sequence and interpatterning. Step 3 represent the ethnographic study of the phenomenon of interest with the goal of understanding systematic context – behavior relationships. Step 4 finally addresses the interpretation of the research findings in relation to the existing research landscape. Based on the research results, existing conceptions and theories can be evaluated.

Although change seems to be an arduous task, scholars should not lapse into lethargy. The complex situation calls for a systematic plan. Kim Bard and colleagues have proposed five steps to make developmental science more inclusive (Bard et al., 2021; Bard et al., 2026). The five steps include: cultural conscious understanding of the context of the phenomenon that should be studied, contextualizing the course of development, arriving at an understanding of the phenomenon that is both inclusively defined and applicable, using the proposed design to investigate developmental phenomena across multiple, diverse samples, and avoiding bias.

In the following, a slightly modified version of four steps is presented:

DOI: 10.4324/9781003672050-20

16.1 Step 1

The process starts with a contextual analysis of the phenomenon of interest: how is the phenomenon defined, who is involved, and where and how is it situated? For example, when attachment is the phenomenon of interest, it is crucial to know: how a baby's social environment looks like, who interacts with a baby, who is responsible for the baby's well-being, what behaviors are displayed with babies, which places are considered appropriate for babies, what the ethnotheories are about children's proper development, what role do relationships play in the ethnotheories, what babies' signals of distress are, how babies are comforted, etc. If ethnographic reports exist about the particular cultural group, it is helpful and advantageous. New contextual information can be extracted from open qualitative interviews, e.g., with cultural informants such as midwives, pediatricians, child care professionals, and, more generally people who are considered culturally competent, but also from mothers belonging to the defined cultural group. The interviews can be conducted with individuals or groups (e.g., focus groups). Local expertise is crucial in evaluating observations. On the other hand, a view from outside and questions from an outsider can help to become aware of the invisible obvious of locals.

Another important avenue is in situ observations, e.g., spot observations (Rogoff, 1978). Yet the meaning of observations needs to be culturally validated, because the same behavior can be interpreted very differently by different cultural groups (Keller, 2022a; de Barbaro & Fausey, 2022; Yahalom & Fein, 2025). Thus, an inclusive approach excludes the application of WEIRD-based instruments in non-WEIRD environments without substantial content-based revision. Even if instruments are adapted, e.g., through language or customization of objects, the culturally relevant dimensions may be missed. For example, if I only look at the mother's presence or absence, the importance of people other than the mother may be missed. If only face-to-face contact is noted, bodily regulations may not be registered. Only by worldwide in situ pilot studies can it be secured that the relevant dimensions are tackled.

16.2 Step 2

The second step consists of studying the developmental course of the phenomenon of interest. It cannot be assumed that the course and the sequence of developmental achievements are the same across cultural environments. Since cultural emphases differ, the timing of developmental achievements differs as well. Therefore, the relationships between developmental achievements, or the interpatterning, may also be different. Moreover, developmental achievements cannot be predicted from the same parameters across cultural environments, nor can developmental achievements have the same consequences across cultural environments. In our research program, we studied developmental tasks that can be assumed to occur in all cultural environments, like self-recognition and autobiographical memory, which nevertheless demonstrated culture-specific phenotypical appearances, developmental courses, and interpatternings (see Keller & Kärtner, 2013, for detailed analysis). We must recognize that there are multiple narratives of human development.

16.3 Step 3

The third step consists of ethnographic studies of the particular phenomenon in defined ecocultural contexts. In our research program, we defined sociodemographic contexts (level of formal schooling, age at first birth, number of children, household composition) as the unit of analysis. These sociodemographic contexts can be compared within and across countries and societies. This way, general contextual adaptations can be identified, which can serve as the basis for general statements. Deviations from the general patterns can be individually explored. In our research program, we identified a general relationship between rural subsistence-based farming cultures and proximal parenting (body contact and body stimulation). Yet, in rural Indian Gujarati farming villages, we found substantially less body contact than expected. It was quite obvious that young Indian Gujarati mothers couldn't carry infants constantly because their body constitution was frail (underweight, anemic). They helped with replacements, e.g., by placing the infants in an old sari, whose two ends were fixed to the ceiling. The cloth wrapped the infants closely through the infants' weight, which was considered to be similar to bodily wrapping (see Keller, 2022a).

16.4 Step 4

The fourth step concerns the evaluation of the research findings within the local meaning systems. The WEIRD mindset with explicit or implicit bias is often used as the default, and local strategies are evaluated as deficiencies. This is probably the most difficult step because it affords a complete paradigm shift in recognizing one's own or learned worldview as one among other equally valid worldviews. One important dimension here is the temporal situatedness of the individual. The WEIRD worldview is based on future orientation, whereas the Global South villagers mostly live in the here and now of the present. This can be observed in diverse areas. For example, WEIRD mothers' conversations with their small babies often concern the future, like "what do you want to do tomorrow?", "should we visit grandma tomorrow?", and "what did daddy tell you yesterday?". Of course, babies' future perspective is still narrow (Demuth et al., 2011). Another example is Martin Daly and Margo Wilson's, the founders of evolutionary psychology, research on future discounting in Brazilian slums, indicating that immediate rewards over larger future ones are preferred as an adaptive response to high-risk environments or low life expectancy (Daly & Wilson, 2005). Also, parenting interventions are aimed at accumulating children's later cognitive capital ("reaching the full developmental potential") through home stimulation and schooling in line with the WEIRD worldview, whereas village life in the Global South is aimed at supporting actual communal coping strategies.

The reevaluation of the research results serves as the basis for deconstructing existing theories. It is a matter of discussion whether, at this point of knowledge accumulation, generating general theories is helpful at all, because the knowledge base is still small. The leading principles must be inclusivity and diversity.

Of course, formulating those strategies (see also Bard et al., 2021, 2026) is not self-sufficient in order to initiate change. They need to become alive in research and practice.

17
OUTLOOK

Throughout the chapters of this book, the problematic knowledge base of developmental psychology and attachment theory, and their applications in particular, has been illuminated. It has been demonstrated that there are substantial flaws in the scientific foundations and a remarkable ignorance of existing evidence from ethnographic research. The reason for this situation has been located in structural and psychological reasons. Ayoto (2025, https://ayoto.substack.com/p/attachment-theory-is-white-supremacy?) talks about the "fantasy of white normativity" that comes under the "guise of scientific objectivity".

It is time for a paradigm shift. The paradigm shift needs to be based on equal collaboration of WEIRD researchers and researchers from the Global South. Establishing research networks on these premises is crucial. National and private funding agencies should set up programs for those networks. Another important step is to include the critical evaluation and concerns of WEIRD theories and conceptions in the teaching curricula at universities and training programs. Curricula need to include cultural consciousness as a taken-for-granted issue of psychology (and the social sciences in general), and ethnography and qualitative methods need to become a natural part of any basic and advanced training so that the parallel worlds of mainstream and critical voices become one. Familiarity can be a first step in changing minds. An example has been proposed by the Past President of the Society for the Teaching of Psychology (Division 2 of the American Psychological Association), Linda Woolf. She created a task force to assemble a repository of resources and materials aimed at decolonizing approaches to teaching and learning in introductory psychology courses and to formulate mandatory standards on these premises (https://teachpsych.org/DecolonizingIntroPsych).

DOI: 10.4324/9781003672050-21

Present times are promising for such a major paradigm shift because critical awareness about the shortcomings, injustice, and ethnocentricity with all the consequences of mainstream research and practice is on the rise.

It is about time that Matsumoto's (2001) prediction that cross-cultural psychology of that time ceased to exist in the 21st century, since it becomes mainstream, has to become reality.

REFERENCES

Abels, M., Keller, H., Mohite, P., Mankodi, H., Shastri, J., Bhargava, S., Jasrai, S., & Lakhani, A. (2005). Early socialization contexts and social experiences of infants in rural and urban Gujarat, India. *Journal of Cross-Cultural Psychology, 36*(6), 717–738.

Abimbola, S. (2024). The foreign gaze: Essays on global health, IRD. https://www.nature.com/articles/d44148-025-00390-0 (retrieved 23.02.2026).

Abimbola, S. (2025). Unawareness, or what we do not (want to) know. In F. L. Jephcott, H. A. Hillary, & C. McGuire (Eds.), *Epidemiological obfuscation. Historical and contemporary case studies*. Abingdon: Routledge Publishers, pp. 233–263.

Abimbola, S., van de Kamp, J., Lariat, J., Rathod, L., Klipstein-Grobusch, K., van der Graaf, R., & Bhakuni, H. (2024). Unfair knowledge practices in global health: A realist synthesis. *Health Policy and Planning, 39*(6), 636–650. https://doi.org/10.1177/1359104520925888

Ainsworth, M. D. S. (1967). *Infancy in Uganda: Infant care and the growth of love*. Baltimore, MD: John Hopkins Press.

Ainsworth, M. D. S., & Marvin, R. S. (1995). On the shaping of attachment theory and research. An interview with Mary D.S. Ainsworth (Fall 1994). *Monographs of the Society for Research in Child Development, 60*(2/3), 2–21.

Ainsworth, M. S., Blehar, M. C., Waters, E., & Wall, S. (1978). *Patterns of attachment: A Psychological study of the strange situation*. Oxford: Lawrence Erlbaum.

Alber, E. (2004). The real parents are the foster parents': Social parenthood among the Baatombu in Northern Benin. In F. Bowie (Ed.), *Cross-cultural approaches to adoption*. Oxfordshire: Routledge, pp. 53–67.

Alter, O. P. M., & Raphael, M. (2024). "I'm always fighting the Coronavirus because it's dangerous to my family": Children's agency, resilience, and role in the family during COVID-19 in Israel. *Developmental Psychology*. Advance online publication. https://doi.org/10.1037/dev0001884

Amici, F., Bietti, L. M., & Liebal, K. (2026, in press). Culturally biased norms, discriminatory outcomes: Why development must go WILD. Comment to Bard,

K. A., Keller, H., & Leavens, D. Let's go WILD: Increasing inclusivity in theories of developmental psychology. *Behavioral and Brain Science, 49*, e259. doi:10.1017/S0140525X25104147.

Anastasi, A. (1958). Heredity, environment, and the question "how?" *Psychological Review, 65*(4), 197–208. 49, e259. doi:10.1017/S0140525X25104147

Arnett, J. (2008). The neglected 95%: Why American psychology needs to become less American. *American Psychologist, 63*(7), 602–614. https://doi.org/10.1037/0003-066X.63.7.602

Bard, K. A., Keller, H., & Leavens, D. (2026). Let's go WILD: Increasing inclusivity in theories of developmental psychology. *Behavioral and Brain Sciences, 49*, e258. doi: 10.1017/S0140525X25000044.

Bard, K. A., Keller, H., Ross, K., Hewlett, B., Butler, L., Boysen, S. T., & Matsuzawa, T. (2021). Joint attention in human and chimpanzee infants in varied socio-ecological contexts. *Monographs of the Society for Research in Child Development, 86*(4), Serial No. 343, 7–217. https://doi.org/10.1111/mono.12435

Barker, R. G. (1965). Explorations in ecological psychology. *American Psychologist, 20*(1), 1–14. https://doi.org/10.1037/h0021697

Barker, R. G., & Wright, H. (1955). *Midwest and its children. The psychological ecology of an american town.* New York: Harper & Row.

Barlow, K. (2001). Working mothers and the work of culture in a Papua New Guinea Society. *Ethos, 29*(1), 78–107.

Barlow, K. (2013). Attachment and culture in Murik society: Learning autonomy and interdependence through kinship, food, and gender. In N. Quinn, & J. Mageo (Eds.), *Attachment reconsidered: cultural perspectives on a Western theory.* New York: Palgrave Macmillan, pp. 165–188.

Barongo-Muweke, N. (2016). *Decolonizing education. Towards reconstructing a theory of citizenship education for postcolonial Africa.* New York: Springer.

Battiste, M. (2017). *Decolonizing education. Nourishing the learning spirit.* Vancouver: UBC Press, Purich Publishing.

Becke, S. D., & Bongard, S. (2018). Comparing attachment networks during middle childhood in two contrasting cultural contexts. *Frontiers in Psychology, 9*(1201). doi: 10.3389/fpsyg.2018.01201

Belsky, J., Steinberg, L., & Draper, P. (1991). Childhood experience, interpersonal development, and reproductive strategy: An evolutionary theory of socialization. *Child Development, 62*(4), 647–670.

Berry, J. W. (2018). Ecocultural perspective on human behavior. In A. K. Üskül, & S. Oishi (Eds.), *Socio-economic and human psychology: Social, ecological, and cultural perspectives.* Oxford: Oxford University Press, pp. 3–33. Retrieved July 20, 2026, from https://doi.org/10.1093/oso/9780190492908.003.0001

Berry, J. W. (2022). Family and youth development: Some concepts and findings linked to ecocultural and acculturation models. *Societies, 12*(6), 181. https://doi.org/10.3390/soc12060181

Bhatia, S., Fernández, J. S., & Sonn, C. C. (Eds.). (2025). *Decolonial psychology. Academic and activist perspectives.* New York: Routledge.

Bischof, N. (1985). *Das Rätsel Ödipus. Die biologischen Wurzeln des Grundkonfliktes von Intimität und Autonomie* (The Oedipus Miracle. Biological roots of the basic conflict between intimacy and autonomy). München: Pieper Verlag.

Bischof-Köhler, D. (2011). *Von Natur aus Anders* (Different by nature). Stuttgart: Kohlhammer–Verlag.

Bjorklund, D. F. (2026, in press). Shared intentionality and attachment theories in WILD and WEIRD contexts. Comment to Bard, K.A., Keller, H., & Leavens, D. (2026, in press). Let's go WILD: Increasing inclusivity in theories of developmental psychology. *Behavioral and Brain Sciences, 49*, e261. https://doi.org/10.1017/S0140525X25104019

Black, M. M., Walker, S. P., Fernald, L. C. H., Andersen, C. T., DiGirolamo, A. M., Lu, C., McCoy, D. C., Fink, G., Shawar, Y. R., Shiffman, J., Devercelli, A. E., Wodon, Q. T., Vargas-Barón, V., Grantham-McGregor, S., for the Lancet Early Childhood Development Series Steering Committee. (2017). Early childhood development coming of age: Science through the life course. *The Lancet, 389*(10064), 77–90.

Bledsoe, C., & Isiugo-Abanihe, U. (1989). Strategies of child fosterage among Mende Grannies in Sierra Leone. In R. Lesthaeghe (Ed.), *Reproduction and social organization in sub-Saharan Africa*. Berkeley: University of California Press, pp. 442–474.

Blum, D. (2002). *Love at Goon Park: Harry Harlow and the science of affection*. New York: Perseus.

Bond, M. H. (2013). Refining Lewin's formula: A general model for explaining situational influence on individual social behavior. *Asian Journal of Social Psychology, 16*(1), 1–15. https://doi.org/10.1111/ajsp.12012

Bowlby, J. (1951). *Maternal care and mental health*. World Health Organization Monograph Series No. 2. Geneva: WHO.

Bowlby, J. (1958). The nature of the child's tie to his mother. *International Journal of Psycho-Analysis, 39*, 350–373.

Bowlby, J. (1969). *Attachment and loss: Volume 1: Attachment*. London: Hogarth Press.

Bowlby, J. (1980). By ethology out of psycho-analysis: An experiment in interbreeding. *Animal Behavior, 28*, 649–656.

Bowlby, J. (1986). *The nature of the child's tie to his mother*. New York: New York University Press.

Brady, I. (Ed.). (2019). *Transactions in kinship: Adoption and fosterage in Oceania*. Honolulu: University of Hawai'i Press.

Branco, A. (2007). Cultural complexities and scientific development. *Integrative Psychological and Behavioral Science, 41*, 41–49. https://doi.org/10.1007/S12124-007-9012-0

Bretherton, I. (1992). The origins of attachment theory. John Bowlby and Mary Ainsworth. *Developmental Psychology, 28*, 759–775.

Britto, P. R., Lye, S. J., Proulx, K., Yousafzai, A. K. Matthews, S. G., Vaivada, T., Perez-Escamilla, R., Rao, N., Ip, P., Fernald, L. C. H., MacMillan, H., Hanson, M., Wachs, T. D., Yao, H., Yoshikawa, H., Cerezo, A., Leckman, J. F., Bhutta, Z. A., Early Childhood Development Interventions Review Group, for the Lancet Early Childhood Development Series Steering Committee. (2017). Nurturing care: Promoting early childhood development. *The Lancet, 389*(10064), 91–102.

Broesch, T., Lew-Levy, S., Kärtner, J., Kanngiesser, P., & Kline, M. (2022). A roadmap to doing culturally grounded developmental science. *Review of Philosophy and Psychology, 14*(2), 587–609. https://doi.org/10.1007/s13164-022-00636-y

Bronfenbrenner, U. (1977). Toward an experimental ecology of human development. *American Psychologist, 32*(7), 513–531. https://doi.org/10.1037/0003-066X.32.7.513

Bronfenbrenner, U., & Evans, G. W. (2000). Developmental science in the 21st century: Emerging questions, theoretical models, research designs and empirical findings. *Social Development, 9*(1), 115–125.

Cadman, T., Diamond, P. R., & Fearon, P. (2017). Reassessing the validity of the attachment Q-sort: An updated meta-analysis. *Infant and Child Development, 27*(1), e2034. https://doi.org/10.1002/icd.2034

Cahan, E. D., & White, S. H. (1992). Proposals for a second psychology. *American Psychologist, 47*, 224–235. https://doi.org/10.1037/0003-066X.47.2.224

Carsten, J. (1995). The substance of kinship and the heat of the hearth: Feeding, personhood, and relatedness among Malays in Pulau Langkawi. *American Ethnologist, 22*(2), 223–241.

Cassidy, J. (2016). The nature of the child's tie. In J. Cassidy, & P. R. Shaver (Eds.), *The handbook of attachment: Theory, research, and clinical applications*. New York: Guilford Press, pp. 3–24.

Cassidy, J., & Shaver, P. R. (2016). *The handbook of attachment: Theory, research, and clinical applications*. New York: Guilford Press.

Chakraborty, S. (2022). *The journey of a mother*. Pune: Vishwakarma Publications.

Chaudhary, N. (2004). *Listening to culture: Constructing reality from everyday talk*. Delhi: Sage Publications.

Chaudhary, N. (2011). Peripheral lives, central meanings: Women and their place in Indian society. In A. C. Bastos, K. Uriko, & J. Valsiner (Eds.), *Cultural dynamics of women's lives*. Charlotte, NC: Information Age, pp. 7–30.

Chen, F., Liu, G., & Mair, C. A. (2011). Intergenerational ties in context: Grandparents caring for grandchildren in China. *Social Forces, 90*(2), 571–594. https://doi.org/10.1093/sf/sor012

Cheung, F. (2012). Mainstreaming culture in psychology. *American Psychologist* (November), *67*(8), 721–730. https://doi.org/10.1037/A0029876

Chisholm, J. S. (1999). *Death, Hope and sex. Steps to an evolutionary ecology of mind and morality*. Cambridge, MA: Cambridge University Press.

Cicchetti, D., & Rogosch, F. A. (1996). Equifinality and multifinality in developmental psychopathology. *Development and Psychopathology, 8*, 597–600.

Cole, M. (1996). *Cultural psychology: A once and future discipline*. Cambridge, MA: Harvard University Press.

Colen, C. G., & Ramey, D. M. (2014). Is breast truly best? Estimating the effects of breastfeeding on long-term child health and wellbeing in the United States using sibling comparisons. *Social Science and Medicine, 109*, 55–65.

Dagan, O., & Sagi-Schwartz, A. (2018). Early attachment network with mother and father. An unsettled issue. *Child Development Perspectives, 12*(2), 115–121.

Dagan, O., Groh, A. M., Madigan, S., & Bernard, K. A. (2021). Lifespan development theory of insecure attachment and internalizing symptoms: Integrating meta-analytic evidence via a testable evolutionary mis/match hypothesis. *Brain Science, 11*(9), 1226. https://doi.org/10.3390/brainsci11091226. Erratum in: *Brain Science*, 2022, *12*(7), 820.

Daly, M., & Wilson, M. (2005). Carpe diem: Adaptation and devaluing the future. *The Quarterly Review of Biology, 89*(1), 55–60.

de Barbaro, K., & Fausey, C. M. (2022). Ten lessons about Infants' everyday experiences. *Current Directions in Psychological Science, 31*(1), 28–33. https://doi.org/10.1177/09637214211059536

De Villiers, S. (2011). *Mothering as a three-generational process: The psychological experience of low-income mothers sharing childcare with their mothers* (Doctoral dissertation). University of Stellenbosch, South Africa.

De Waal, F. B. M. (2001). *The ape and the sushi master: Cultural reflections of a primatologist*. New York: Basic Books.

De Wolff, M., & van IJzendoorn, M. (1997). A meta-analysis on parental antecedents of infant attachment. *Child Development, 68*, 571–591.

DeJesus, J. M., Callman, M. A., Soliss, G., & Gelman, S. A. (2019). Generic language in scientific communication. *Proceedings of the National Academy of Sciences, 116*(37), 18370–18377.

Demuth, C., Keller, H., Gudi, H., & Otto, H. (2011). Developmental precursors of autonomy and relatedness: Discursive practices in childhood and autobiographical self-constructions in young adulthood. In K. Jensen de López, & T. G. B. Hansen (Eds.), *Development of self in culture in mind. Vol. 1: Self in culture in mind*. Aalborg, DK: Aalborg University Press, pp. 89–119.

Diamond, J. (2013). *The world until yesterday*. New York: Penguin Books.

Diamond, J., & Robinson, J. A. (2010). *Natural experiments of history*. Harvard: Harvard University Press.

Dirie, W. (1999). *Desert flower*. New York: William Morrow Paperbacks.

Dollberg, D., & Keren, M. (2020). Factors contributing to continuity and discontibuity in child psychopathology from infancy to childhood: An explorative study. *Clinical Child Psychology and Psychiatry, 25*(4), 891–908. https://doi.org/10.1177/1359104520925888

Doyle Jr., J. (2007). Child protection and child outcomes: Measuring the effects of foster care. *American Economic Review, 97*(5), 1583–1610.

Duschinsky, R. (2020). *Cornerstones of attachment research*. Oxford: Oxford University Press.

Duschinsky, R. (2025). Sheri Madigan and the determinants of child development lab, calgary. *Developments in Attachment Research, 1* (Oxford, 2025; online ed, Oxford Academic, 2 June 2025). https://doi.org/10.1093/9780191976643.003.0005, accessed 13.08.2025.

Duschinsky, R., Bakkum, L., Mannes, J. M. M., Skinner, G. C. M., Turner, M., Mann, A., Coughlan, C., Reijman, S., Foster, S., & Beckwith, H. (2021). Six attachment discourses: Convergence, divergence and relay. *Attachment & Human Development, 23*(4), 355–374. https://doi.org/10.1080/14616734.2021.1918448

Eibl-Eibesfeldt, I. (2004). *Die Biologie des menschlichen Verhaltens: Grundriss der Humanethologie* (Biology of human behavior. Outline of human ethology) (5 ed.). Vierkirchen-Pasenbach: Blank Media.

Else-Quest, N. M., Hyde, J. S., & Clark, R. (2003). Breastfeeding, bonding, and the mother-infant relationship. *Merrill-Palmer Quarterly, 49*(4), 495–517.

Engle, P. L., Black, M. M., Behrman, J. R., Cabral de Mello, M., Gertler, P. J., Kapiriri, L., Martorell, R., Young, M. E., & International Child Development Steering Group. (2007). Strategies to avoid the loss of developmental potential in more than 200 million children in the developing world. *The Lancet, 369*(9557), 229–242.

Fearon, P. R., & Schuengel, C. (2021). What kinds of relationships count as attachment relationships? In R. A. Thompson, J.-A. Simpson, & L. J. Berlin (Eds.), *Attachment: The fundamental questions*. New York: Guilford, pp. 24–30.

Fearon, R. P., Bakermans-Kranenburg, M. J., van IJzendoorn, M. J., Lapsley, A., & Roisman, G. I. (2010). The significance of insecure attachment and disorganization in the development of children's externalizing behavior: A metanalytic study. *Child Development, 81*, 435–456.

Fonseca, C. (2004). The circulation of children in a Brazilian working-class neighborhood: A local practice in a globalized world. In F. Bowie (Ed.), *Cross-cultural approaches to adoption*. Oxfordshire: Routledge, pp. 185–201.

Forslund, T., Granqvist, P., van IJzendoorn, M., Sagi-Schwartz, A., Glaser, D., Steele, M., Hammarlund, M., Schuengel, C., Bakermans-Kranenburg, M. J., Steele, H., Shaver, P. R., Lux, U., Simmonds, J., Jacobvitz, D., Groh, A. M., Bernard, K., Cyr, C., Hazen, N. L., Foster, S.,… Duschinsky, R. (2021). Attachment goes to court: Child protection and custody issues. *Attachment & Human Development, 24*(1), 1–52.

Foster, S. L., Schofield, G., Geoghegan, L., Hood, R., Sagi-Schwartz, A., Bakkum, L., … Duschinsky, R. (2025). Attachment theory and research: What should be on the core curriculum for child and family social workers? *Social Work Education, 45*(3), 803–820. https://doi.org/10.1080/02615479.2025.2531859

Fox Keller, E. (2010). *The mirage of a space between nature and nurture.* Durham, NC: Duke University Press.

Funk, L., Scheidecker, G., Chapin, B. L., Schmidt, W. J., El Quardani, C., & Chaudhary, N. (2023). *Feeding, bonding and the formation of social relationships.* Cambridge: Cambridge Elements.

Gaskins, S., Beeghly, M., Bard, K. A., Gernhardt, A., Liu, C. H., Teti, D. M., Thompson, R. A., Weisner, T. S., & Yovsi, R. D. (2017). Meaning and methods in the study and assessment of attachment. In H. Keller, & K. A. Bard (Eds.), *The cultural nature of attachment: Contextualizing relationships and development.* Cambridge: MIT Press, pp. 195–229.

Geangu, E., Bengo, O., Stahl, D., & Striano, T. (2010). Contageous crying beyond the first days of life. *Infant Behavior and Development, 33*(3), 279–288.

Gernsbacher, M. A., Akhtar, N., & Dinishak, J. (2026). An inclusive developmental science requires attention to neurodiversity. Comment to Bard, Keller & Leavens. Let' s go Wild: Increasing inclusivity in theories of developmental psychology. *Behavioral and Brain Sciences, 49*, e268. doi: 10.1017/S0140525X25104020

Gijsbers, B., Mesters, I., Knottnerus, A. J., Legtenberg, A. H., & van Schayck, C. P. (2005). Factors influencing breastfeeding practices and postponement of solid food to prevent allergic disease in high-risk children: Results from an explorative study. *Patient Education and Counseling, 57*(1), 15–21.

Gilkerson, J., Richards, J. A., Warren, S. F., Montgomery, J. K., Greenwood, C. D., Oller, D. K., Hansen, J. H. L., & Paul, T. D. (2017). Mapping the early language environment using all – Day recordings and automated analysis. *American Journal of Speech-Language Pathology, 26*(2), 248–265. https://doi.org/10.1044/2016_AJSLP-15-0169

Görlitz, D., Harloff, H. J., Mey, G., & Valsiner, J. (Eds.). (1998). *Children, cities, and psychological theories. Developing relationships.* Berlin: de Gruyter.

Gottlieb, A. (2004). *The afterlife is where we come from: The culture of infancy in West Africa.* Chicago, IL: University of Chicago Press.

Gottlieb, A. (2014). Is it time to detach from attachment theory? Perspectives from the West African rain forest. In O. Otto, & H. Keller (Eds.), *Different faces of attachment: Cultural variations on a universal human need.* Cambridge: Cambridge University Press, pp. 187–214.

Gould, S. J. (1996). *Full house: The spread of excellence from Plato to Darwin.* New York: Harmony Books.

Granqvist, P., Sroufe, L. A., Dozier, M., Hesse, E., Steele, M., van IJzendoorn, M., Solomon, J., Schuengel, C., Fearon, P., Bakermans-Kranenburg, M., Steele, H., Cassidy, J., Carlson, E., Madigan, S., Jacobvitz, D., Foster, S., Behrens, K., Rifkin-Graboi, A., Gribneau, N., Ward, M. J., … Duschinsky, R. (2017).

Disorganized attachment in infancy: A review of the phenomenon and its implications for clinicians and policy-makers. *Attachment & Human Development, 19*(6), 534–558. https://doi.org/10.1080/14616734.2017.1354040
Grantham-McGregor, S., Chang, S. M., Smith, J. A., Dunkelberg, E., Rubio-Codina, M., & Walker, S. P. (2024). Theory, principles and key content of the Reach Up Curriculum. doi: 10.1044/2016_AJSLP-15-0169
Gratier, M. (2003). Expressive timing and interactional synchrony between mothers and infants. Cultural similarities, cultural differences, and the immigration experience. *Cognitive Development, 8*(4), 533–554.
Greenfield, P. M., & Keller, H. (2004). Cultural psychology. In C. Spielberger (Ed.), *Encyclopedia of applied psychology*. Oxford: Elsevier, pp. 545–553.
Grossmann, K. E., Grossmann, K., Huber, F., & Wartner, U. (1981). German children's behavior towards their mothers at 12 months and their fathers at 18 months in Ainsworth's strange situation. *International Journal of Behavioral Development, 4*(2), 157–181.
Guthrie, R. V. (1976). *Even the rat was white. A historical view of psychology*. New York: Allyn & Bacon Classic Edition.
Harkness, S., Super, C., & van Tien, N. (2000). Individualism and the "western mind" reconsidered: American and Dutch parents' ethnotheories of the child. *New Directions in Child and Adolescence Development, 87*, 23–39. https://doi.org/10.1002/cd.23220008704
Harlow, H. F., & Zimmermann, R. R. (1959). Affectional responses in the infant monkey. *Science, 130*(3373), 421–432.
Hart, B., & Risley, T. R. (1992). American parenting of language-learning children: Persisting differences in family-child interactions observed in natural home environments. *Developmental Psychology, 28*, 1096–1105. https://doi.org/10.1037/0012-1649.28.6.1096
Hart, B., & Risley, T. R. (1995). *Meaningful differences in the everyday experience of young American children*. Baltimore, MD: Brookes.
Hart, B., & Risley, T. R. (2003). The early catastrophe. *Education Review, 17*, 110–118.
Hart, J. (2006). Saving children: What role for anthropology? *Anthropology Today, 22*(1), 5–8.
He, J., & Van de Fijver, F. (2012). Bias and equivalence in cross-cultural psychology. *Online Readings in Psychology and Culture, 2*(2). https://doi.org/10.9707/2307-0919.1111
Heft, H. (2001). *Ecological psychology in context: James Gibson, Roger Baker and the legacy of William James's radical empiricism*. New York: Psychology Press.
Henrich, J., Heine, S. J., & Norenzayan, N. (2010). The weirdest people in the world? *Behavioral and Brain Sciences, 33*(2–3), 61–83.
Hewlett, B. S. (1991). *Intimate fathers: The nature and context of Aka Pygmy paternal infant care*. Ann Arbor: University of Michigan Press.
Hewlett, B. S., Lamb, M. E., Shannon, D., Leyendecker, B., & Schölmerich, A. (1998). Culture and early infancy among central African foragers and farmers. *Developmental Psychology, 34*(4), 653–661. https://doi.org/10.1037/0012-1649.34.4.653
Hinde, R. A. (1982). Attachment: Some conceptual and biological issues. In C. Murray Parkes, & J. Stevenson-Hinde (Eds.), *The place of attachment in human behavior*. New York: Basic Books, pp. 60–76.
Houghtaling, B., Shanks, C. B., Ahmed, S., & Rink, E. (2018). Grandmother and health care professional breastfeeding perspectives provide opportunities for

health promotion in an American Indian community. *Social Science & Medicine, 208*, 80–88.

Howes, C. (2009). Friendship in early childhood. In W. M. Bukowski, B. Laursen, & K. H. Rubin (Eds.), *Handbook of peer interactions, relationships, and groups.* New York: Guilford, pp. 180–194.

Isiugo-Abanihe, U. C. (1985). Child fosterage in West Africa. *Population and Development Review, 11*(1), 53–73.

Jahoda, G. (2012). Critical reflections on some recent definitions of "culture". *Culture & Psychology, 18*(3), 289–303. https://doi.org/10.1177/1354067X12446229

Janowski, N., & Kerlogue, F. (2007). *Kinship and food in south east Asia.* Copenhagen: Nias Press.

Jansen, J., de Weerth, C., & Riksen-Walraven, J. M. (2008). Breastfeeding and the mother-infant relationship: A review. *Developmental Review, 28*(4), 503–521.

Juffer, F., Bakermans-Kranenburg, M. J., & Van IJzendoorn, M. H. (2023). *Promoting positive parenting. An attachment based intervention.* New York: Routledge.

Jukes, M. C. H., Zuilkowski, S. s., & Grigorenko, E. (2018). Do schooling and urban residence develop cognitive skills at the expense of social responsibility? A study of adolescence in the Gambia, West Africa. *Journal of Cross – Cultural Psychology, 49*(1), 82–98.

Kabeer, N. (2024). *Renegotiating patriarchy: Gender, agency and the Bangladesh paradox.* London: LSE Press.

Kagan, J., & Snidman, N. (2004). *The long shadow of temperament.* Cambridge, MA: Harvard University Press.

Kagitcibasi, C. (2017). *Family, self and human development across cultures: Theory and applications.* New Work: Routledge Classic Edition.

Karen, R. (1994). *Becoming attached: First relationships and how they shape our capacity to love.* New York: Oxford University Press.

Kärtner, J., Keller, H., Chaudhary, N., & Yovsi, R. (Eds.). (2012). The development of mirror self-recognition in different socio-cultural contexts. *Monographs of the Society for Research in Child Development, 77*(4), Serial-No. 305, 1–87.

Keller, H. (2000). Evolutionary approaches to the life span. In A. L. Comunian, & U. P. Gielen (Eds.), *Cross-cultural perspectives on human development.* Padua: Cedam, pp. 117–130.

Keller, H. (2004). Adventures in research. Field studies and their challenges. *Cross-Cultural Psychology Bulletin, 38*(1, 2), 6–9.

Keller, H. (2007). *Cultures of infancy.* Mahwah, NJ: Erlbaum. (2022) New York: Routledge Classic Edition.

Keller, H. (2010). The motorische Entwicklung aus kulturvergleichender Perspektive (Motor development from an cross-cultural perspective). In I. Hunger, & R. Zimmer (Eds.), *Bewegte Kindheit.* Schorndorf: Verlag Hofmann, pp. 23–43.

Keller, H. (2012a). Autonomy and relatedness revisited: Cultural manifestations of universal human needs. *Child Development Perspectives, 6*(1), 12–18. https://doi.org/10.1111/j.1750-8606.2011.00208.x

Keller, H. (2012b). Die Autonomieillusion. Kindheit in Deutschland zwischen Anspruch und Wirklichkeit (The illusion of autonomy. Childhood in Germany between entitlement and reality). In R. Braches-Chyrek, C. Röhner, & H. Sünker (Eds.), *Kindheiten. Gesellschaften. Interdisziplinäre Zugänge zur Kindheitsforschung.* Leverkusen: Barbara Budrich, pp. 205–223.

Keller, H. (2017). Cultural and historical diversity in early relationships formation. *European Journal of Developmental Psychology, 05*, 700–713.

Keller, H. (2019). The role of emotion in socialization processes across cultures: Implications for theory and practice. In D. Matsumoto, & H. C. Hwang (Eds.), *The handbook of culture and psychology*. New York: Oxford University Press, pp. 209–234.

Keller, H. (2022a). *The myth of attachment theory*. London: Routledge.

Keller, H. (2022b). Mentalisierung aus Kulturvergleichender Perspektive (Mentalizing from a cross–cultural perspective). In H. Kirsch, T. Nolte, & S. Gingelmaier (Eds.), *Soziales Lernen, Beziehung und Mentalisierung*. Böhlau: Vandenhoeck & Ruprecht, pp. 62–75.

Keller, H., & Bard., K. A. (Eds.). (2017). *The cultural nature of attachment: Contextualizing relationships and development*. Cambridge: MIT Press.

Keller, H., & Chaudhary, N. (2017). Is the mother essential for attachment? Models of care in different cultures. In H. Keller, & K. A. Bard (Eds.), *The cultural nature of attachment: Contextualizing relationships and development*, Strüngmann Forum Reports. Cambridge: MIT Press, pp. 109–138.

Keller, H., & Demuth, C. (2005). Further explorations of the "Western mind". Mothers' and grandmothers' parental ethnotheories in Los Angels, California, and Berlin, Germany. *Forum Qualitative Social Research, 7*(1), Art. 5. https://www.qualitative-research.net/index.php/fqs/article/view/74/151, retrieved 8.1.2013.

Keller, H., & Greaves, M. (2016). Karibisch Kochen (3rd ed.). Berlin: edition diá.

Keller, H., & Kärtner, J. (2013). Development. The cultural solution of universal developmental tasks. In M. Gelfand, C. Y. Chiu, & Y. Y. Hong (Eds.), *Advances in culture and psychology*, Vol. 3. New York: Oxford University Press, pp. 63–116.

Keller, H., & Otto, H. (2009). The cultural socialization of emotion regulation during infancy. *Journal of Cross-Cultural Psychology, 40*(6), 996–1011.

Keller, H., Yovsi, R. D., & Voelker, S. (2002). The role of motor stimulation in parental ethnotheories. The case of Cameroonian Nso and German women. *Journal of Cross-Cultural Psychology, 33*(4), 398–414.

Keller, H., Yovsi, R. D., Borke, J., Kärtner, J., Jensen, H., & Papaligoura, Z. (2004). Developmental consequences of early parenting experiences: Self regulation and self recognition in three cultural communities. *Child Development, 75*(6), 1745–1760.

Kerlogue, F. (2007). Food and the family: Assimilation in a Malay village. In M. Janowski, & F. Kerlogue (Eds.), *Kinship and food in southeast Asia*. Copenhagen: Nias Press, pp. 54–70.

Kessel, F. (Ed.). (2025). *Pillars of developmental psychology. Recollections and reflections*. New York: Cambridge University Press.

Klaus, M. H., & Kennell, J. H. (1976). *Maternal – Infant bonding: The impact of early separation and loss on family development*. St. Lois: Mosby.

Kline, M. A., Shamsudheen, R., & Broesch, T. (2018). Variation in the universal: Making cultural evolution work in developmental psychology. *Philosophical Transactions of the Royal Society B, 373*(1743), 20170059. https://doi.org/10.1098/rstb.2017.0059

Kowitz, P. (2023). Rethinking the principle of Parens Patriae: Ther Aria Shah case from a cultural and child rights perspective. *Institutionalised Children Explorations and Beyond*, 1–16. https://doi.org/10.1177/23493003231207149

Kroeber, A. L., & Kluckhohn, C. (1952). *Culture: A critical review of concepts and definitions – The history of human culture, its role in social sciences*. Philadelphia, PA: Pantianos Classics.

Kronborg, H., Harder, I., & Hall, E. O. (2015). First time mothers' experiences of breastfeeding their newborn. *Sexual & Reproductive Healthcare, 6*(2), 82–87.

Kroupin, I., Davis, H. E., & Henrich, J. (2025). Beyond Newton: Why assumptions of universality are critical to cognitive science, and how to finally move past them. *Psychological Review, 132*(2), 291–310. https://doi.org/10.1037/rev0000480

Lamm, B., Schmidt, W. J., Ndzenyuiy, M. N., & Keller, H. (2023). Growing up in Nso: Changes and continuities ion children's relational networks during the first three years of life. *Ethos, 51*(1), 27–46.

Lancy, D. (2022). *The anthropology of childhood: Cherubs, chattel, changelings* (3rd ed.). Cambridge: Cambridge University Press.

Lancy, D. F. (2016). Playing with knives: The socialization of self-initiated learners. *Child Development, 87*(3), 654–665. https://doi.org/10.1111/cdev.12498

Lavelli, M., Carra, C., Rossi, G., & Keller, H. (2019). Culture-specific development of early mother-infant emotional co-regulation: Italian, Cameroonian, and West African immigrant dyads. *Developmental Psychology, 55*(9), 1850–1867. https://doi.org/10.1037/dev0000696

Leiderman, P. H., & Leiderman, G. F. (1974). *Familial influences on infant development in an East African agricultural community*. Oxford: John Wiley & Sons.

Leinaweaver, J. (2014). Informal kinship-based fostering around the world: Anthropological findings. *Child Development Perspectives, 8*(3), 131–136.

Leung, F. M. (2012). Mainstreaming culture in psychology. *American Psychologist, 67*(8), 721–730. https://doi.org/10.1037/a0029876

LeVine, R. A., Dixon, S., LeVine, S., Keefer, C. H., Richman, A., Leiderman, P. H., & Brazelton, T. B. (1994). *Child care and culture: Lessons from Africa*. Cambridge: Cambridge University Press. https://doi.org/10.1017/CBO9780511720321

Levins, R., & Lewontin, R. (1985). *The dialectical biologist*. Boston, MA: Harvard University Press.

Levit, G. S., Meister, K., & Hoßfeld, U. (2008). Alternative evolutionary theories: A historical survey. *Journal of Bioeconomics, 10*, 71–96. https://doi.org/10.1007/s10818-008-9032-y

Lewin, K. (1935). *A dynamic theory of personality*. New York: McGraw.

Linde, K., Lehnig, F., Nagl, M., & Kersting, A. (2020). The association between breastfeeding and attachment: A systematic review. *Midwifery, 81*, 102592. https://doi.org/10.1016/j.midw.2019.102592

Liu, F., Wang, Y., Wang, N., Ye, Z., & Fang, S. (2023). Embracing the Ebb and flow of life: A latent profile analysis of impermanence and its association with mental health outcomes among Chinese university students. *Mindfulness, 14*(9), 2224–2235. https://doi.org/10.1007/s12671-023-02213-5

Lopez, A. E., & Singh, H. (2024). *Decolonizing educational knowledge: International perspectives and contestations*. London: Palgrave Macmillan.

Main, M., & Solomon, J. (1986). Discovery of an insecure-disorganized/disoriented attachment pattern. In T. Brazelton, T. Berry, & M. W. Yogman (Eds.), *Affective development in infancy*. New York: Ablex Publishing, pp. 95–124.

Marks, A. K., & Garcia-Coll, C. (2012). *The immigrant paradox in children and adolescents: Is becoming American a developmental risk*? New York: American Psychological Association. https://doi.org/10.1037/13094-000

Markus, H. R., & Schwartz, B. (2010). Does choice mean freedom and well-being. *Journal of Consumer Research, 37*(2), 344–355.

Marvin, R. S., Van Devender, T. L., Iwanaga, M. I., LeVine, S. & LeVine, R. A. (1977). Infant-caregiver attachment among the Hausa in Nigeria. In H. McGurk (Ed.), *Ecological factors in human development*. Amsterdam: North Holland, pp. 247–260.

Matsumoto, D. (2001). Cross-cultural psychology in the 21st century. In J. S. Halonen, & S. F. Davis (Eds.), *The many faces of psychological research in the 21st century* (chapter 5). Retrieved from the Society for the Teaching of Psychology Web site: https://teachpsych.org/ebooks/faces/index_faces.php

Mayr, E. (1988). *Towards a new philosophy of biology*. Cambridge, MA: Harvard University Press.

McGoey, L. (2012). Strategic unknowns: Towards a sociology of ignorance. *Economy and Society, 4*(1), 1–16.

McGoey, L. (2019). *The unknowers: How strategic ignorance rules the world*. London: ZED Books Ltd.

Mead, M. (1954). Some theoretical considerations on the problem of mother-child separation. *American Journal of Orthopsychiatry, 24*(3), 471–483. https://doi.org/10.1111/j.1939-0025.1954.tb06122.x

Meehan, C. L., & Hawks, S. (2013). Cooperative breeding and attachment among the Aka Foragers. In N. Quinn, & J. M. Mageo (Eds.), *Attachment reconsidered: Cultural perspectives on a Western theory*. New York: Palgrave Macmillan, pp. 85–113.

Melhuish, E., Ereky-Stevens, K., Petrogiannis, K., Ariescu, A., Penderi, E., Rentzou, K., Tawell, A., Slot, P., Broekhuizen, M., & Leserman, P. (2015). A review of research on the effects of early childhood education and care (ECEC) on child development. In *Curriculum Quality Analysis and Impact Review of European Early Childhood Education and Care*. CARE - European Early Childhood Education and Care.

Meins, E. (2017). Overrated: The predictive power of attachment. *The Psychologist, 30*, 20–24.

Mesman, J. (2021). Attachment theory's universality claim: Asking different questions. In R. A. Thompson, J. A. Simpson, & L. J. Berlin (Eds.), *Attachment. The fundamental questions*. New York: The Guilford Press, pp. 245–251.

Mesman, J., van Ijzendoorn, M. H., & Sagi-Schwartz, A. (2016). Cross-cultural patterns of attachment. In J. Cassidy, & P. Shaver (Eds.), *The handbook of attachment: Theory, research, and clinical applications*. New York: Guilford Press, pp. 852–877.

Mezzenzana, F. (2023). Amazonian childcare. *Aeon*, 20.06.

Michaelis, R. (2006). *Die ersten fünf Jahre im Leben eines Kindes*. (The first five years in the life of a child). München: Knaur Verlag.

Mikulincer, M., & Shaver, R. S. (2021). The continuing influence of early attachment orientations viewed from a personality – Social perspective on adult attachment. In R. A. Thompson, J. A. Simpson, & L. J. Berlin (Eds.), *Attachment. The fundamental questions*. New York: The Guilford Press, pp. 211–218.

Miller, A. T. (1998). Child fosterage in the United States: Signs of an African heritage. *The History of the Family, 3*(1), 35–62.

Miller, J. G. (1999). Cultural psychology: Implications for basic psychological theory. *Psychological Science, 10*(2), 85–91. https://doi.org/10.1111/1467-9280.00113

Miller, P. J., Sperry, D. E., & Sperry, L. L. (2024). A deficit story in motion: How marginalized youngsters are defined out of the educational game before they enter school. *Journal of Social Issues, 80*, 1218–1237. https://doi.org/10.1111/josi.12647

Mistry, J., Contreras, M., & Dutta, R. (2013). Culture and child development. In R. M. Lerner, M. A. Easterbrooks, J. Mistry, & I. B. Weiner (Eds.), *Handbook of psychology* (2nd ed.) Volume 6, *Developmental psychology*. New York: John Wilesy & Sons, Inc., pp. 265–285.

Moewert, T. (2021). Sie leben nicht von Milch allein. (They do not live only from milk). Hoyersverda: Verlag das netz.

Morelli, G. A. (1987). *A comparative study of Efe (Pygmy) and Lese one-, two- and three-year-olds of the Ituri forest of northeastern Zaire: The influence of subsistence-related variables and children's age and gender on social-emotional development* (Doctoral Dissertation). University of Massachussetts. https://hdl.handle.net/20.500.14394/11420, https://doi.org/10.7275/10879

Morelli, G. A., Quinn, N., Chaudhary, N., Vicedo, M., Rosabal-Coto, M., Keller, H., Murray, M., Gottlieb, A., Scheidecker, G., & Takada, A. (2018). Ethical challenges of parenting interventions in low to middle income countries. *Journal Cross-Cultural Psychology, 49*(1), 5–24. https://doi.org/10.1177/0022022117746241

Moscovici, S. (2000). Social representations. In G. Duveen (Ed.), *Explorations in social psychology*. Cambridge: Polity.

Nadan, Y., & Roer-Strier, D. (2020). A context-informed perspective of child risk and protection: Deconstructing myths in the risk discourse. *Journal of Family Theory & Review, 12*(2), 464–477. https://doi.org/10.1111/jftr.12393.

Ndzenyuiy, M., & Keller, H. (2025). The cultural nature of collaboration. In P. F. M. J. Verschure (Ed.), *Strüngmann forum reports* (Vol. 33). Cambridge: MIT Press, pp. 125–139.

Newson, M., Buhrmester, M., Xygalatas, D., & Whitehouse, H. (2021). Go wild, not weird. *Journal for the Cognitive Science of Religion, 6*(1/2), 80–106. https://doi.org/10.1558/jcsr.38413

NICHD Early Child Care Research Network (2001). Nonmaternal care and family factors in early development: An overview of the NICHD study of early child care. *Journal of Applied Developmental Psychology, 22*, 457–492.

Nielsen, M., Haun, D., Kärtner, J., & Legare, C. H. (2017). The persistent sampling bias in developmental psychology: A call to action. *Journal of Experimental Child Psychology, 162*, 31–38.

Nisbett, R. (2019). *The geography of thought. How Asians and Westeners think differently*. New York: John Murray Business.

Notermans, C. (2004). Fosterage and the politics of marriage and kinship in East Cameroon. In F. Bowie (Ed.), *Cross-cultural approaches to adoption*. Oxfordshire: Routledge, pp. 68–83.

Nsamenang, A. B. (1992). Perceptions of parenting among the Nso of Cameroon. In B. S. Hewlett (Ed.), *Father-child relations: Cultural and biosocial contexts*. Hawthorn, NY: Aldine, pp. 321–343.

Nsamenang, A. B. (2007). *Human development in cultural context*. New York: Sage.

Ochs, E., & Kremer-Sadlik, T. (2020). Ethical blind spots in ethnographic and developmental approaches to the language gap debate. *Langage et société, 2*(170), 39–67.

Oppong, S. (2015). A critique of early childhood development research and practice in Africa. *Africanus, 45*(1), 23–41.

Oppong, S. (2019). Overcoming obstacles to a truly global psychological theory, research, and praxis in Africa. *Journal of Psychology in Africa, 29*(4), 292–300.

Oppong, S. (2023). Epistemological allyship. *Psychology and Developing Societies , 35*(1), 69–86.

Oppong, S., & Strader, S. (2022). *Interventions that matter start with local cultures: Issues and strategies in early childhood care and education interventions in Africa.* An ECCE Project Supported by Spencer Foundation/Boston College.

Otto, H. (2014). Don't show your emotions! Emotion regulation and attachment in the Cameroonian Nso. In H. Otto, & H. Keller (Eds.), *Different faces of attachment. Cultural variations of a universal human need.* Cambridge: Cambridge University Press, pp. 215–229.

Otto, H., & Keller, H. (Eds.). (2014) *Different faces of attachment. Cultural variations of a universal human need.* Cambridge: Cambridge University Press.

Packer, M. J. (2026). *Child development. Understanding a cultural perspective.* New York: Sage.

Peñacoba, C., & Catala, P. (2019). Associations between breastfeeding and mother–infant relationships: A systematic review. *Breastfeeding Medicine, 14*(9), 616–629.

Quinn, N. (2013). Adult attachment cross-culturally: A reanalysis of the Ifaluk emotion Fago. In N. Quinn, & J. Mageo (Eds.), *Attachment reconsidered.* New York: Palgrave Macmillan, pp. 215–239.

Quinn, N., & Mageo, J. M. (Eds.). (2013). *Attachment reconsidered: Cultural perspectives on a Western theory.* Basingstoke: Palgrave Macmillan/Springer Nature. https://doi.org/10.1057/9781137386724

Rabain-Jamain, J. (2001). Language use in mother-child and young sibling interactions in senegal. *First Language, 21*(63), 357–385. https://doi.org/10.1177/014272370102106307

Robinson, W. (1950). Ecological correlations and the behavior of individuals. *American Sociological Review, 75*, 351–357.

Roer-Strier, D., & Nadan, Y. (Eds.). (2020). *Context-informed perspectives of child risk and protection in Israel.* New York: Springer.

Rogoff, B. (1978). Spot observation: An introduction and examination. *Quarterly Newsletter of the Institute for Comparative Human Development, 2*(2), 21–26.

Rogoff, B. (2003). *The cultural nature of human development.* Oxford: Oxford University Press.

Rogoff, B., & Chavajay, P. J. (1995). What's become of research on the cultural basis of cognitive development? *American Psychologist, 50*(10), 859–877. https://doi.org/10.1037/0003-066X.50.10.859

Rogoff, B., & Mejía-Arauz, R. (2022). The key role of community in *Learning by Observing and Pitching In* to family and community endeavours. *Journal for the Study of Education and Development, 45*(3), 494–548. https://doi.org/10.1080/02103702.2022.2086770

Roisman, G. I., & Groh, M. (2021). The legacy of early attachments. Past, present, future. In R. A. Thompson, J. A. Simpson, & L. J. Berlin (Eds.), *Attachment. The fundamental questions.* New York: Guilford Press, pp. 187–194.

Rosabal-Coto, M., Quinn, N., Keller, H., Vicedo, M., Chaudhary, N., Gottlieb, A., Scheidecker, G., Murray, M., Takada, A., & Morelli, G. A. (2017). Real-world applications of attachment theory. In H. Keller, & K. A. Bard (Eds.), *The cultural nature of attachment: Contextualizing relationships and development*. Cambridge: MIT Press, pp. 335–354.

Rosenfeld, S. (2025). *The age of choice: A history of freedom in modern life*. Princeton, NJ: Princeton University Press.

Salinas, D. A., Fouts, H. N., Neitzel, C. L., & Bates-Fredi, D. R. (2019). Young children's social networks in an informal urban settlement in Kenya: Examining network characteristics among Kamba, Kikuyu, Luo, and Maasai children. *Journal of Cross-Cultural Psychology, 50*(5), 639–658.

Sanches de Oliveira, G., & Baggs, E. (2023). *Psychology's WEIRD problems*. Boston, MA: Cambridge University Press.

Sánchez-Mira, N., & Saura, D. M. (2020). Attachment parenting among middle-class couples in Spain: Gendered principles and labor divisions. *Journal of Family Studies, 28*(2), 1–18.

Saraswathi, T. S., & Pai, S. (1997). Socialization in the Indian context. In H. S. R. Kao, & D. Sinha (Eds.), *Asian perspectives on psychology*. New Delhi: Sage, pp. 74–92.

Scheidecker, G. (2023). Parents, caregivers, and peers: Patterns of complementarity in the social world of children in rural Madagascar. *Current Anthropology, 64*(3), 286–320.

Scheidecker, G. (2025). *Beyond parents: The social world of early childhood and its developmental significance*. Cham: Palgrave Macmillan.

Scheidecker, G., Chaudhary, N., Keller, H., Mezzenzana, F., & Lancy, D. (2023). Poor brain development in the global south: Challenging the evidence base of early childhood interventions. *Ethos, 51*(1), 3–26.

Scheidecker, G., Chaudhary, N., Oppong, S., Röttger-Rössler, B., & Keller, H. (2022). Different is not deficient: Respecting diversity in early childhood development. *The Lancet Child & Adolescent Health, 6*(12), E24–E25.

Scheler, M. (2018). *Die Stellung des Menschen im Kosmos* (The position of humans in Cosmos). Hamburg: Felix Meiner Verlag.

Schmidt, W. J., Keller, H., & Rosabal-Coto, M. (2023a). The cultural specificity of parent – Infant interactions: Perspectives of urban middle – Class and rural indigenous families in Costa Rica. *Infant Behavior and Development, 70*, 101796. https://doi.org/10.1016/j.infbeh.2022.101796

Schmidt, W. J., Keller, H., Rosabal-Coto, M., Fallas Gamboa, K., Solís Guillén, C., Durán-Delgado, E. (2023b). Feeding, food, and attachment: An underestimated relationship? *Ethos, 51*(1), 1–19. https://doi.org/10.1111/etho.12380

Schmied, V., & Lupton, D. (2001). Blurring the boundaries: Breastfeeding and maternal subjectivity. *Sociology of Health & Illness, 23*(2), 234–250.

Schröder, L., Keller, H., Kärtner, J., Kleis, A., Abels, M., Yovsi, R. D., Chaudhary, N., Jensen, H., & Papaligoura, Z. (2013). Early reminiscing in cultural context: Cultural models, maternal reminiscing styles, and children's memories. *Journal of Cognition and Development, 14*(1), 10–34.

Schuengel, C., de Schipper, J. C., Sterkenburg, P. S., & Kef, S. (2013). Attachment, intellectual disabilities and mental health: Research, assessment and intervention. *Journal of Applied Research of Intellectual Disabilities, 26*(1), 34–46. https://doi.org/10.1111/jar.12010. PMID: 23255377.

Sears, W., & Sears. M. (2001). The attachment parenting book. New York: Little, Brown & Company.

Semrau, K. E. A., Hirschhorn, L. R., Marx Delaney, M., Singh, V. P., Saurastri, R., Sharma, N., Tuller, D. E., Firestone, R., Lipsitz, S., Dhingra-Kumar, N., Kodkany, B. S., Kumar, V., Gawande, A. A., & BetterBirth Trial Group. (2017). Outcomes of a coaching-based WHO safe childbirth checklist program in India. *New England Journal of Medicine, 377*(24), 2313–2324. doi: 10.1056/NEJMoa1701075

Semrau, K. E. A., Miller, K. A., Lipsitz, S., Fisher-Bowman, J., Karlage, A., Neville, B. A., Krasne, M. et al. 2020. Does adherence to evidence-based practices during childbirth prevent perinatal mortality? A post-hoc analysis of 3,274 births in Uttar Pradesh, India. *BMJ Global Health, 5*(9), e002268.

Serpell, R. (2011). Social responsibility as a dimension of intelligence, and as an educational goal: Insights from programmatic research in an African society. *Child Development Perspectives, 5*(2), 126–133.

Serpell, R., & Nsamenang, A. B. (2014). Locally relevant and quality ECCE programmes: Implications of research on indigenous African child development and socialization. *Early Childhood Care and Education Working Papers Series, 3*. Paris: UNESCO(ED.2013/WS/38).

Sewell, W. H. (2023). The concept(s) of culture. In *Beyond the cultural turn: New directions in the study of society and culture*. Berkeley: University of California Press, pp. 35–61. https://doi.org/10.1525/9780520922167-003

Seymour, S. C. (2013). 'It takes a village to raise a child': Attachment theory and multiple child care in Alor, Indonesia, and in North India. In N. Quinn, & J. Mageo (Eds.), *Attachment reconsidered*. New York: Palgrave Macmillan, pp. 115–139.

Shweder, R. A., & Bourne, E. J. (1984). Does the concept of a person vary cross-culturally? In R. A. Shweder, & R. A. LeVine (Eds.), *Culture theory: Essays on mind, self and emotion*. Cambridge, MA: Cambridge University Press, pp. 158–199.

Singh, L. (2024). Decolonizing and diversifying research in cognitive development. *Journal of Cognition and Development, 25*(2), 175–179. https://doi.org/10.1080/15248372.2024.2324000

Singh, M. (2025). Medical benchmarks and the myth of the universal patient. *The New Yorker*, 03.31.

Slabu, L., Lenton, A. P., Sedikides, C., & Bruder, M. (2014). Trait and state authenticity across cultures. *Journal of Cross - Cultural Psychology, 45*(9), 1347–1373.

Smith, L. T. (1999). *Decolonizing methodologies: Research and Indigenous peoples*. London: ZED Books.

Sperry, D. E., Sperry, L. L., & Miller, P. J. (2018). Reexamining the verbal environments of children from different socioeconomic backgrounds. *Child Development, 90*, 1303–1318. https://doi.org/10.1111/cdev.13072

Stern, E. (2023). Research on intelligence and learning: How to unite estranged siblings. *Personality and Individual Differences, 221*, 112555.

Stone, J., Smith, H. T., & Murphy, L. B. (Eds.). (1973). *The competent infant: Research and commentary*. New York: Routledge.

Super, C. M., & Harkness, S. (1996). The cultural structuring of child development. In J. W. Berry, P. R. Dasen, & T. S. Saraswathi (Eds.), *Handbook of cross-cultural psychology, Vol. 2: Basic processes and human development* (2nd ed.). Boston, MA: Allyn & Bacon, pp. 1–39.

Sweis, R. K. (2021). *Paradoxes of care. Children and global medical aid in Egypt*. Stanford, CA: Stanford University Press.

Syed, M. (2026, in press). Psychology wants to stay WEIRD, not go WILD. Commentary to Bard et al. Let' s go WILD: Increasing inclusivity in theories of developmental psychology. *Behavioral and Brain Sciences*, *49*, e278. doi: 10.1017/S0140525X25104172

Taras, V., & Steel, P. (2009). Beyond Hofstede: Challenging the ten commandments of cross-cultural research. In C. Nakata (Ed.), *Beyond Hofstede: Culture frameworks for global marketing and management*. Basingstoke: Macmillan/Palgrave, pp. 40–60.

Thalmayer, A. G., Toscanelli, C., & Arnett, J. J. (2025).The neglected 95% revisited: Is American psychology becoming less American? *American Psychologist, 76*(1), 116–129.

Thompson, R. A. (2026). Embracing diversity for a reason. Embracing behavioral diversity for a reason. *Behavioral and Brain Sciences*, *49*, e279. doi:10.1017/S0140525X25104093

Thompson, R. A. (2017). Twenty-first century attachment theory: Challenges and opportunities. In H. Keller, & K. A. Bard (Eds.), *The cultural nature of attachment*. Cambridge: MIT Press, pp. 301–320.

Thompson, R. A., Braun, K., Grossmann, K. E., Gunnar, M. R., Heinrichs, M., Keller, H., O'Connor, T. G., Spangler, G., Voland, E., & Wang, S. (2005). Group report: Early social attachment and its consequences. The dynamics of a developing relationship. In C. S. Carter, L. Ahnert, K. E. Grossmann, M. E. Lamb, S. B. Hrdy, S. W. Porges, & N. Sachser (Eds.), *Attachment and bonding. A new synthesis*. New York: MIT Press, pp. 349–383.

Thompson, R. A., Simpson, J. A., & Berlin, L. J. (2022). Taking perspective on attachment theory and research: Nine fundamental questions. *Attachment & Human Development, 24*(5), 543–560. https://doi.org/10.1080/14616734.2022.2030132

Thorndike, E. (1939). On the fallacy of imputing the correlations found for groups to the individuals or smaller groups composing them. *American Journal of Psychology, 52*(1), 122–124.

Tooby, J., & Cosmides, L. (1992). The psychological foundations of culture. In J. H. Barkow, L. Cosmides, & J. Tooby (Eds.), *The adapted mind: Evolutionary psychology and the generation of culture*. Oxford: Oxford University Press, pp. 19–136.

Toomela, A., & Valsiner, J. (Eds.). (2010). *Methodological thinking in psychology. 60 years gone astray?* Charlotte, NJ: Information Age Publishing Inc.

Triandis, H. C. (2007). Culture and psychology: A history of the study of their relationship. In S. Kitayama, & D. Cohen (Eds.), *Handbook of cultural psychology*. New York: The Guilford Press, pp. 59–76.

Tronick, E. Z., Morelli, G. A., & Ivey, P. K. (1992). The Efe Forager infant and Toddler's pattern of social relationships: Multiple and simultaneous. *Developmental Psychology, 28*(4), 568–577.

Tronick, E. Z., Morelli, G. A., & Winn, S. (1987). Multiple caretaking of Efe (Pygmy) infants. *American Anthropologist, 89*(1), 96–106.

True, M. M., Pisani, L., & Oumar, F. (2001). Infant–mother attachment among the Dogon of Mali. *Child Development, 72*(5), 1451–1466.

Tsai, J. L., Miao, F. F., Seppala, E., Fung, H. H., & Yeung, D. Y. (2007). Influence and adjustment goals: Sources of cultural differences in ideal affect. *Journal of Personality and Social Psychology, 92*(6), 1102–1117. https://doi.org/10.1037/0022-3514.92.6.1102

Tuli, M., & Chaudhary, N. (Eds.). (2025). *Reframing developmental psychology. Perspectives from the global South*. Leeds: Emerald Publishing.

Tuli, M., & Negi, B. (Eds.). (2025). *Ethical considerations for research and practice in the human sciences*. Charlotte: IAP. ISBN 979-8-88730-863-0. https://tinyurl.com/322ehc4y

Üskül, A. K., Kitayama, S., & Nisbett, R. E. (2008). Ecocultural basis of cognition: Farmers and fishermen are more holistic than herders. *PNAS, 105*(25), 8552–8556. https://doi.org/10.1073/pnas.0803874105

van den Boom, D. C. (1994). The influence of temperament and mothering on attachment and exploration: An experimental manipulation of sensitive responsiveness among lower-class mothers with irritable infants. *Child Development, 65*(5), 1457–1477. https://doi.org/10.1111/j.1467-8624.1994.tb00829.x

van den Boom, D. C. (1997). Sensitivity and attachment: Next steps for developmentalists. *Child Development, 68*(4), 592–594. PMID: 9306637.

Van der Horst, F. C. P. (2011b). Mary Ainsworth's role in the study of attachment. In F. C. P. Van der Horst (Ed.), *John Bowlby – From psychoanalysis to ethology: Unraveling the roots of attachment theory*. New York: Wiley, pp. 131–153. https://doi.org/10.1002/9781119993100.refs

Van der Horst, F. C. P. (Ed.). (2011a). *John Bowlby – From psychoanalysis to ethology: Unraveling the roots of attachment theory*. New York: Wiley https://doi.org/10.1002/9781119993100.ch6, 08.09.2018.

van IJzendoorn, M. H., & Sagi-Schwartz, A. (2008). Cross-cultural patterns of attachment. Universal and contextual dimensions. In J. Cassidy, & P. Shaver (Eds.), *Handbook of attachment. Theory, research and clinical applications*. New York: Guilford Press, pp. 880–905.

Varnum, M. E., Grossmann, I., Kitayama, S., & Nisbett, R. E. (2010). The origin of cultural differences in cognition: Evidence for the social orientation hypothesis. *Current Directions in Psychological Science, 19*(1), 9–13. https://doi.org/10.1177/0963721409359301

Verhage, M. L., Schuengel, C., Madigan, S., Fearon, R. M. P., Oosterman, M., Cassibba, R., Bakermans-Kranenburg, M. J., & van IJzendoorn, M. H. (2016). Narrowing the transmission gap: A synthesis of three decades of research on intergenerational transmission of attachment. *Psychological Bulletin, 142*(4), 337–366. https://doi.org/10.1037/bul0000038

Verhoef, H. (2005). A child has many mothers': Views of child fostering in Northwestern Cameroon. *Childhood, 12*(3), 369–390.

Vicedo, M. (2013). *The nature and nurture of love: From imprinting to attachment in cold war America*. Chicago, IL: University of Chicago Press.

Vicedo, M. (2017a). Putting attachment in its place: Disciplinary and cultural contexts. *European Journal of Developmental Psychology, 14*(6), 684–699. https://doi.org/10.1080/17405629.2017.1289838, 08.09.2018.

Vicedo, M. (2017b). The strange situation of the ethological theory of attachment: A historical perspective. In H. Keller, & K. A. Bard (Eds.), *The cultural nature of attachment*. Cambridge: MIT Press, pp. 13–52.

Vicedo, M. (2018). On the history, present, and future of attachment theory, reply to Duschinsky, van IJzendoorn, Foster, Reijman & Lionetti attachment histories and futures. *European Journal of Developmental Psychology, 17*(1), 147–155. https://doi.org/10.1080/17405629.2018.1502920.

Voland, E. (1993). *Grundriss der Soziobiologie* (Outline of sociobiology). Heidelberg and Berlin: Spektrum Akademischer Verlag.

Walker, S. P., Wachs, T. D., Grantham-McGregor, S., Black, M. M., Nelson, C. A. Huffman, S. L., Baker-Henningham, H., Chang, S. M., Hamadani, J. D., Lozoff, B., Gardner, J. M. M., Powell, C. A., Rahman, A., & Richter, L. (2011). Inequality in early childhood: Risk and protective factors for early child development. *The Lancet, 378*(9799), 1325–1338. doi: 10.1016/S0140-6736(11)60555-2

Walmsley, E. (2008). Raised by another mother: Informal fostering and kinship ambiguities in northwest Ecuador. *Journal of Latin American and Caribbean Anthropology, 13*(1), 168–195.

Waters, E., & Deane, K. E. (1985). Defining and assessing individual differences in attachment relationships: Q-methodology and the organization of behavior in infancy and early childhood. In I. Bretherton, & E. Waters (Eds.), *Monographs of the Society for Research in Child Development*, vol. 50, nos. 1–2, pp. 41–65.

Weber, A., Fernald, A., & Diop, Y. (2017). When cultural norms discourage talking to babies: Effectiveness of a parenting program in rural Senegal. *Child Development, 88*(5), 1513–1526.

Weisner, T. S. (2002). Ecocultural understanding of children's developmental pathways. *Human Development, 45*(4), 275–281.

Weisner, T., S., & Gallimore, R. (1977). My brother's keeper: Child and sibling caretaking. *Current Anthropology, 18*(2), 169–190.

Whiting, B. B. (1980). Culture and social behavior: A model for the development of social behavior. *Ethos, 8*, 95–116.

Whiting, B. B., & Edwards, C. P. (1988). *Children of different worlds. The formation of social behavior.* Cambridge, MA: Harvard University Press.

Whiting, B. B., & Whiting, J. W. M. (1975). *Children of six cultures: A psychocultural analysis.* Cambridge, MA: Harvard University Press.

Whiting, J. W. M. (1977). A model for psychocultural research. In P. Leiderman, S. Tulkin, & A. Rosenfeld (Eds.), *Culture and infancy.* New York: Academic Press, pp. 29–47.

Wierzbicka, A. (1990). The meaning of colour terms: Semantics, culture, and cognition. *Cognitive Linguistics, 1*(1), 99–150.

Wiggins, B. J., & Christopherson, C. D. (2019). The replication crisis in psychology: An overview for theoretical and philosophical psychology. *Journal of Theoretical and Philosophical Psychology, 39*(4), 202–217. https://doi.org/10.1037/teo0000137

Wilkinson, R. B., & Scherl, F. B. (2006). Psychological health, maternal attachment and attachment style in breast- and formula-feeding mothers: A preliminary study. *Journal of Reproductive and Infant Psychology, 24*(1), 5–19.

Wober, M. (1972). Culture and the concept of intelligence: A case in Uganda. *Journal of Cross - Cultural Psychology, 3*(3), 327–328. https://doi.org/10.1177/002202217200300312

Worthman, C. M. (2016). Ecocultural theory: Foundations and applications. In C. M. Hay (Ed.), *Methods that matter: Integrating mixed methods for more effective social science research.* Chicago, IL: University of Chicago Press, online edn. https://doi.org/10.7208/chicago/9780226328836.003.0002

Wrigley, E. A., & Hutchinson, S. A. (1990). Long-term breastfeeding: The secret bond. *Journal of Nurse-Midwifery, 35*(1), 35–41.

Yahalom, J., & Fein, E. (2025). Fostering cultural engagement through ethnographic psychological research: An introduction to the special section. *Qualitative Psychology, 12*(1), 25–33. https://doi.org/10.1037/qup0000327

Yovsi, R. D. (2003). *Ethnotheories about breastfeeding and mother-infant interaction: The case of sedentary Nso farmers and nomadic Fulani pastorals with their infants 3–6 months of age in Mbven sub division of the northwest province of Cameroon*. Münster: LIT Verlag.
Yovsi, R. D., & Keller, H. (2007). The architecture of cosleeping among wage-earning and subsistence farming Cameroonian Nso families. *Ethos, 35*(1), 65–84.
Yovsi, R. D., & Keller, K. (2003). Breastfeeding: An adaptive process. *Ethos, 31*(2), 147–171.
Zentner, M. (2025). Reflexionen zu drei prägenden Prämissen der Bindungsforschung (Reflections to three formative premises of attachment research). *Familiendynamik, 50*(3), 206–218.

INDEX

Note: *Italic* page numbers refer to figures and page numbers followed by "n" denote endnotes.